Conquering the Giants

Foreword

Numbers 13, an Old Testament book of the Bible, tells the story of a man named Caleb. The title of this book, <u>Conquering the Giants</u>, is based on that man's story.

After miraculously freeing the Israelites from their long years of captivity in Egypt, God led them across the desert towards a land He promised to give them. When they arrived at their destination, twelve spies went in to scope out the land. They saw a wonderful land filled with milk and honey, but they also saw giant men that inhabited the land. They knew they would have to fight for their inheritance.

When the spies reported back about what they had observed, ten of them fearfully announced there was no way they could conquer this beautiful land because they felt the Israelites were "like grasshoppers compared to those men". However, two of the spies, Caleb and Joshua, boldly reminded the Israelites that it didn't matter about their size or that they were outnumbered. With faith and pride, they stalwartly proclaimed with God on their side, they would *conquer the giants*! Caleb wasn't intimidated by worldly impossibilities. He knew His God was more powerful than any force that stood against them. If God promised them they would have this land, then God would help them overcome any obstacle to make sure He kept His word.

My son, Caleb, has had many challenges. He also has had to face many "giants" – from major brain damage to negligent medical care and much more. However, against all odds, with God's intervention, he has conquered these giants.

Like the ancient Caleb of the Bible, my son Caleb's story is one where God gets the glory for overcoming seemingly impossible obstacles!

Acknowledgements

First and foremost, I want to thank God who actually wrote this story long before Caleb even existed. I simply have had the honor of narrating His good works. However, I do want to thank Ann Berkley for giving me the idea to actually write down this glorious story. Secondly, I want to thank my good friends – Alepha Khonga, Jackie Cooper, and Debi Howell – who willingly sacrificed their time to read my book and offer wonderful editing suggestions. Last but not least, I want to thank my husband who patiently played with the kids so I could write on his rare days off or he went to bed alone and endured the noise of the typing of keys late into the night as I wrote. I love you Percy and think you are the most amazing man on the planet! I am so thankful that God blessed me to walk this journey of life by your side!

Table of Contents

Chapter One

Our world turns upside down

Ouch! I felt a tight pain in my stomach. It was Sunday, September 6, 2009, around 8:00 at night in the capital city of Gaborone, located in the country of Botswana on the continent of Africa. Nine months of my second healthy pregnancy were predicted to end on September 9, 2009. If this was labor, our baby had made it full term and almost to his due date.

AUGH! There it was again. Was it real labor or just those Braxton Hicks contractions? Immediately, I told my husband, Percy, to get out the stopwatch. Trying not to get too excited, we recognized a pattern. The pains were coming about every two minutes and lasting about 30-45 seconds. Visions of holding our little baby boy in my arms began to flash across my mind. Could tonight be the night? Was the long wait over? Would tomorrow be the day our small family of three become a family of four? I could visualize the little body cuddling up to me and falling asleep against my chest. I could imagine his little fingers grasping tightly around mine as I pictured myself gazing down at his tiny features.

We waited another hour just to be sure. Finally, we couldn't deny it any longer; the contractions weren't letting up. Surely we were going to meet Caleb, our little boy whom we had talked to, dreamed of, and prayed for countless times over the past year! We called our neighbor who had agreed to look after our daughter, Anna Catherine, when I went into labor. By eleven o'clock that night, all our bags were packed. We could barely contain our excitement as we quietly picked up our 22-month-old sleeping daughter from her bed. Though I was in pain, the joy of knowing what was coming gave me the strength to hold her as my husband drove the short distance to our neighbor's house. We gently placed her in bed and quietly whispered in her ear, "When you wake up tomorrow, you will finally meet your baby brother!"

We called my gynecologist on the way and told him I was in labor. We arrived at the hospital around midnight and met him there. After four hours of intense and close contractions, I was hoping to be "half way" there at least. The doctor examined me and said I was only dilated a weak 1 cm. He said if it weren't for the fact that I seemed to be in pain, he would send me home and tell me to come back in the morning. Optimistically, I told him I hoped it would progress faster and would prefer to stay there. He left and told the nurses to call him when I was further along. Eight o'clock the next morning, Monday, September 7, rolled around and I was still at 1 cm. Twelve hours of labor and nothing to show for it! The nurses were getting frustrated with me, as if it were my fault it wasn't progressing! Finally, I couldn't take the pain anymore and asked for pain medication. They said they could only give me pain medication if I was in "real labor". 1 cm. didn't qualify, even though the monitor on my stomach confirmed that hard contractions were coming every two minutes! Around ten o'clock that morning, they finally conceded and gave me an epidural which completely numbed me from the pain and provided much wanted relief. I began to dilate a bit but still was not progressing. Throughout the whole labor, the nurses on duty called my gynecologist a couple of times; but he never came back to check on me and assess what was happening. Around two o'clock that afternoon, he showed up. He told me the head of my child hadn't crowned. Although I still had 2 cm. to go until I was fully dilated, he wanted to take the baby out. Then, he pulled out these HUGE metal FORCEPS! Fear gripped me! "*NO, I cried*! Please don't use those! In America, where I am from, I always hear horror stories when those are used!"

He replied with arrogance, "Maybe in America, they don't know how to use them properly, but, in Africa, we have experience. It is perfectly safe. Just relax and trust me." Everything in me screamed NO, but at this point I was just too tired to argue and he seemed so confident it would be fine. My husband, who was helping to support my legs, told me he inserted the forceps and positioned them around little Caleb's head. Next, Percy told me that he put his foot on the bed for "leverage" and pulled with all his might, yanking Caleb's frail little body out of my body by his head.

At 2:44 p.m., Caleb Andrew Thaba entered the world. Weighing 3.5 kg. (7.7 lbs) and being 53 centimeters (21 inches) in length, he looked like any healthy baby boy. But as soon as he was born, my intuition as a mother told me something was wrong. He didn't cry. The doctor kept hitting him on the back … but with no reaction. The nurses whisked him to a table and put an oxygen mask on him. The doctor "cleaned" me up, and the nurses attended to Caleb. No one indicated that anything about Caleb was abnormal so I tried to tell myself I was just imagining things. I told them I wanted to breastfeed him. They handed him to me, but he wouldn't suck. In fact, he lay motionless. He wouldn't even grasp my finger when I put it in his tiny hand. They quickly took him back and told me he would go to the nursery and I should go get some rest. I was assured once I had gotten some sleep they would bring him back to me.

The hospital had strict visiting hours in the maternity ward so my husband had been forced to leave; I was left there all alone. After a couple of hours, I realized I wasn't going to be able to sleep until I knew what was happening with our baby. All I wanted to do was snuggle with our little baby boy. I beckoned a nurse, "Please, can you bring my baby? I would like to try and breastfeed again." She nodded yes and left the room. An hour passed. The nurse didn't return. I was in a room with three other mothers so another nurse came and helped one of the other mothers. I waited until she finished attending her, got her attention and asked her if she could please let me know what was happening with our son. It had been five hours and surely he needed to eat by now! She returned and told me he was sleeping and not to worry. The minutes ticked on. Due to my epidural, my legs still felt like jelly or I would have marched down to the nursery myself! By eleven o'clock that night, I think I had asked all of the nurses on rotation to bring me our baby; but none of them would tell me anything or bring Caleb. It had been nine hours since he was born. I had feeling back in my legs again. I didn't care that I still had the catheter in me and was supposed to lay flat until the doctor came in the morning to take it out of me. I didn't care that due to my stitches and eighteen and a half hours of labor, I was in enormous pain. I WAS DETERMINED TO SEE MY BABY!

I located the nursery. I looked around, and immediately my eyes locked on my son. He was lying in an incubator with oxygen blowing in his face. Sounds of babies crying, babies cooing, and little arms flailing against the tiny beds filled the room. None of these noises came from Caleb. His eyes were open, but he lay perfectly still staring up at the plastic box he was in. I asked the nursery nurse if I could hold him. With a nod, she helped me take him out and positioned him on my chest to breastfeed. He laid there without moving. He wouldn't suck. He didn't cry. He wouldn't grasp my fingers. His limp body just lay lifeless in my arms. With tears, I turned to the nursery nurse and begged her with my eyes to tell me the truth. "What's wrong with him?" I whispered. Again, I was brushed off and told not to worry. This time, I had had enough! I exclaimed, "NO! Something is wrong with my son! I AM worried! Someone needs to tell me what is happening! It has been nine hours and my son hasn't eaten. He should be at the very least crying out of hunger!" She pricked his foot to test his blood sugar and told me he wasn't starving and was probably just exhausted from my long labor. She promised she would call me if he showed any signs of hunger.

Around three o'clock in the middle of the night, she woke me up and said, "I have just changed his diaper; come and try to feed him again". Same story... This time, she said "Okay, I think you should write down your observations and tell the pediatrician tomorrow what you have noticed. Ask him if he is going to run any tests on your son." Mixed emotions filled me. I didn't know whether to be happy that finally someone was starting to act like something was wrong or sad because now I knew for sure that she also had noticed something abnormal.

It was now Tuesday morning, September 8th. At seven o'clock the next morning I went down to the nursery and tried to feed him again...same story. This was now the third time I had tried to feed him in the nursery. I was VERY concerned that it had now been almost seventeen hours and he hadn't eaten anything! Since the nursery was full of babies that needed attention and Caleb wasn't crying, they ignored him. He was the least of their concerns as he lay there not making a sound. I said, "At least, can't you put an i.v. in him or something to give him some nutritional intake?!" She responded that the pediatrician would do his rounds at eight o'clock, an hour from now, and she would be advised of what actions she needed to take then. I was told to go back to my room and rest, assured that everything would be fine.

I limped back and slowly eased my aching body down on the dingy sheets, feeling all alone and helpless. Our baby boy was obviously suffering and there was nothing I could do about it. I knew he wasn't getting adequate medical care. This made me wish I could somehow have gotten to America for his birth. I rolled over and wept, begging God to help my son. I wanted to call Percy, but I knew he also hadn't slept the day before and needed his sleep. I held myself back and just prayed there in that hospital bed in Botswana, Africa so very far from home.

When the doctor made his rounds, he stated that Caleb had vomited meconium and he had advised they pump his stomach and place a drip in his arm to replace his fluids. I listened carefully and then pulled out my list of concerns asking him if he planned on running any tests. He replied, "IF I feel like it!" With a huff, he turned and stormed out of the room! I was stunned! I was speechless! Did he just say that!? I had waited all night to talk to a doctor hoping that finally someone could tell me what was going on, and he acted like I OFFENDED him! WHAT WAS GOING ON!?

As the morning wore on, phone calls of congratulations streamed in. Each time, as my friends' cheerful voices congratulated me on Caleb's birth, I would break out fresh in tears and blubber, "Something is wrong with him." Word began to get out and the tone of the phone calls started changing. With concerned voices, my friends assured me that God was in control and everything would work out. A prayer group from the church came and led me in prayer and again reminded me that God loved me and had a plan for me and baby Caleb.

I sat dazed. It wasn't supposed to be like this. I was supposed to be holding Caleb, gently planting little kisses on his face. He was supposed to be cooing in my arms. I was supposed to be playing with his little toes and tickling his tiny feet. These visits from my friends were supposed to be finding me a proud mom showing off my new little bundle of joy.

When Percy showed up that morning, I fell in his arms weeping. I tried to recount the previous night's events. My husband, always the one to think the best in people and situations, assured me I was just tired and overreacting. Because Caleb was in an incubator, he was confined to the nursery. Men weren't allowed in the nursery so Percy hadn't actually gotten close to Caleb since those five minutes after birth. However, he could peer through the nursery window, and he "looked fine" to him. I felt like I was going mad! Why was everyone downplaying this? I KNEW something was gravely wrong, yet no one would take me seriously!

As the day went on, I remembered something I had read at some point in my life; babies respond positively to touch. I wasn't allowed to hold him on Tuesday, so I forced myself to stand there beside his incubator. I poked my hand through the little plastic hole and lovingly stroked his unresponsive tiny body. The temperature gauge was set so high that beads of sweat rolled from his lifeless body. Continually, I wiped his forehead, changing the drenched paper towel under his head every couple of minutes. "Is this normal?" I inquired of the nurse. Surely, he shouldn't be sweating like this! She assured me that babies need to be hot, and he was okay. I later learned he was being severely dehydrated.

Wednesday morning, September 9th, during the doctors' daily rounds my gynecologist notified me that all looked okay with me. I was set to go home at lunch. Sadly, the pediatrician didn't have such good news. He informed us that Caleb had shown signs of seizures that morning. He explained he wasn't too worried about it, but it was enough of a concern that they should keep him in the hospital a couple of more days. His next statement got me thinking. He suspected my baby had hypoxic ischemic encephaly. In layman's terms, he thought my baby had lost some oxygen in his brain sometime during the pregnancy. In a defensive tone, he quickly added, "It definitely happened during the pregnancy, not during the delivery. For sure, it wasn't caused by the forceps. We just don't know what all happens within your uterus during pregnancy."

Why was he defending that this wasn't caused by the forceps or during delivery? He, the pediatrician, hadn't even been present at the birth. Was he trying to protect the gynecologist? At that point, I hadn't even begun the blame game that this could have been prevented if the doctor wouldn't have used forceps. After he left, I remarked to Percy, "This must have happened during delivery and probably was caused by the forceps!"

Sometime that morning, my pastor's wife came in to visit me. When I reported what was going on, she replied with urgency in her voice to GET OUT of that hospital and get to a hospital in South Africa! Despite all that was happening, I couldn't help but smile. Wasn't that a bit extreme? I mean, yes, I could tell something was wrong, but how do you even go about getting a baby in an incubator to another country!? "No," I replied, "the doctor says it really isn't that big of a deal."

She then took my husband out into the hall and insisted, "Get out of here and get to South Africa. My brother is a pediatric neurologist in Pretoria. I think he can help Caleb. Something about this situation doesn't sound right." My husband also thanked her for her concern but responded it sounded a bit excessive. She wouldn't take no for an answer! Finally, we began to listen.

The morning passed in a blur as my pastor's wife and another church friend quickly helped me prepare for Caleb's emergency evacuation. Percy and

I had to add Caleb's name to our insurance, get a passport for him to cross the border, pack a bag for us to go to South Africa for an indefinite amount of time, arrange babysitters for our daughter who would remain behind for an indefinite amount of time, and call the medical rescue team to arrange an immediate evacuation flight.

Before leaving the hospital, one additional thing needed was a letter from the pediatrician attending Caleb in Botswana to the pediatrician who would receive him in South Africa. He needed to give a report of what had been done and what had happened so far. Since he had told me basically nothing in the past three days, I asked him if I could see a copy of the report. He responded angrily, "That is none of your business!" Honestly, at the time I was so happy that he had agreed to write the report so that we could leave, I didn't complain. After all, he had been so rude to me the entire hospital stay that I was pretty scared of him. But one of my friends from church, who was helping me get ready for the evacuation, was really frustrated by that comment and emphatically exclaimed, "It IS your business what is going on with your son! Make sure you see a copy of that report!"

Finally, Caleb and I were ready. Unfortunately, Percy would have to find his own way. Only mother and child were allowed in the small evacuation plane. The medical rescue men whisked Caleb away from the private hospital in Botswana. People scurried out of the way staring dumbfounded, probably wondering what was so bad that an ambulance would come to take a patient AWAY from a hospital. Following close behind, I overheard the medical rescue men discussing Caleb's vital signs. "The seizures are reoccurring every five minutes." I looked at Caleb and watched as he blinked his eyes fast and bit his lower lip. That was a seizure?! He had been doing that all morning! For the first time, I started to really grasp how serious this was. I am no doctor, but I know having reoccurring seizures every five minutes for a three-day-old baby is NOT good!

When we got on the plane and the medical rescue men opened Caleb's file, I asked sweetly if I could see the report the doctor had denied me access to. Politely, one of the men handed me his file. I was shocked beyond words. The doctor who had assured me on more than one occasion that he was only a "bit concerned" about Caleb, but it was no big deal, had written that his kidneys had shut down yesterday (Tuesday). He was vomiting blood and having reoccurring seizures! He knew it was serious and he hadn't let on at all to me. THANK

GOD for my pastor's wife who had insisted we get out of there! My son was dying in the hospital, and it seemed the doctors weren't planning on doing anything about it!

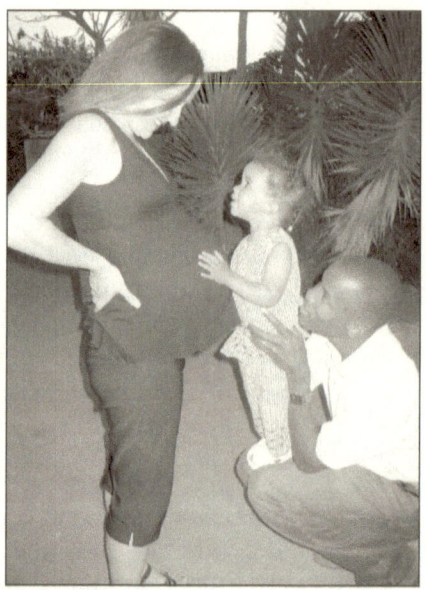

Family picture the day before I went into labor with Caleb

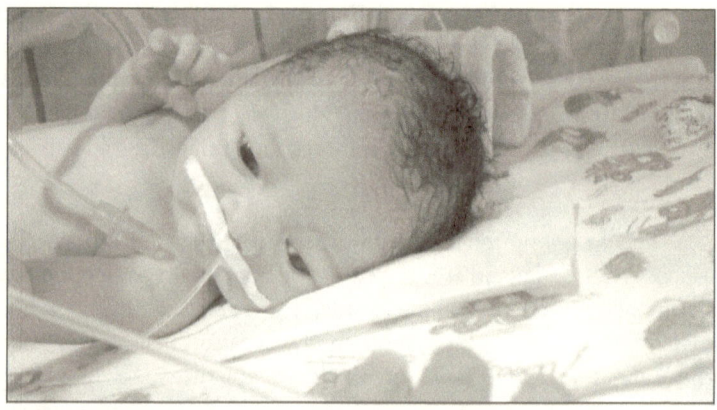

Caleb in the incubator at the private hospital in Botswana

Chapter Two

Thinking back

As I looked out of the airplane window at the clouds passing by, my son lay convulsing an arm's length away. I cried silently out to God. A Bible verse began to run across my mind over and over. It was a passage from John 9. A man had been born blind and some people came to Jesus and said, "Whose sin caused this man to be born blind? Was it his or his parents?" Jesus responded, "Neither, this was done so that the work of God might be displayed in his life." I wasn't sure why or how, but I knew God was telling me that Caleb's life was going to bring Him glory. Somehow the work of God was going to be displayed in Caleb's life. A glimmer of hope poked through the dark cloud that surrounded me. Was God saying He would heal Caleb? I so earnestly wanted to believe that. Instead, the verses that kept coming to my mind were verses of surrender. I was reminded of stories where God got the glory because people chose to praise Him even when they didn't get their way! Was I willing to testify to God's greatness at the end of the day if Caleb died? What if he was severely brain-damaged? Worst-case scenarios paraded through my mind as I asked myself the tough questions of how deep my faith in God ran.

As I sat there gazing out the window, I thought back on my life. What was I, an American lady, doing in Botswana anyway? Why had I chosen to give birth in a third world country?

My mind rolled back to a hot summer's day in Daytona Beach, Florida, when I was a twelve years old. I was on a youth retreat with my church, First Baptist Church of Tifton, Georgia.

Even though, it was over twenty years ago, I remembered it like it was yesterday. Boys spat wadded paper balls through straws. Girls giggled. Some dozed. In spite of the distractions, something in my youth pastor's message gripped me. He quoted Matthew 28:19-20 (NIV): *"Therefore go and make disciples of all nations, baptizing them in the name of the Father and of the Son and of the Holy Spirit, and teaching them to obey everything I have commanded you. And surely I am with you always, to the very end of the age."*

He pointed out that the command is to go, and it is directed to all disciples of Jesus. However, in our world, he noted, most people live in reverse. They stay unless they are "called" to go. He challenged us to plan on GOING unless God specifically called us to stay. He handed out commitment cards, requesting we put it in writing if we were seriously willing to GO and preach the gospel to the nations.

I came home jumping up and down! "I know what I want to be when I grow up," I danced and sang gleefully. "I want to be a missionary in Africa!" At first, I think my parents thought it was a "phase" that I would grow out of as I matured. My father is a lawyer, and my mother has two masters' degrees in school psychology. Being a missionary in Africa probably wasn't in the cards when they had dreamed what their little girl would be when she grew up. But the desire only grew the older I got. Throughout high school, I taught younger Sunday school classes and travelled to numerous foreign countries participating in short term mission trips. In my summers, I volunteered as a summer youth intern in various churches. During my college years, I served as a youth minister at a local church. By the time I was getting ready to graduate, I was confident of my calling. I applied to be a journeyman with the International Mission Board and was accepted into their program. In August of 2000, I moved to Francistown, Botswana for a 2 year term on the "field."

I moved into a secluded house without a phone. My computer broke down with a virus my first week in Francistown, and it took four months to fix it. The street lights barely worked, and my only neighbor was a man who was building his house with bricks he made daily in his yard. He spoke no English. I worked with youth in the secondary schools preaching the gospel and discipling those who wanted to grow in their faith. I had no friends who were my age.

It should have been one of the loneliest times in my life. Instead, it was one of the happiest, most fulfilling experiences of my life. I had NOTHING but Jesus to live for! The Lord blessed my ministry, and I saw many come to know Jesus. Daily, I was filled with such gratitude that God would consider me worthy to be used by Him. I had to pinch myself because life was so marvelous! Did I really get paid to do that which my heart deeply desired to do anyway? Was it really my JOB to go out and tell people Jesus loved them and had a plan for them? My inner joy and peace confirmed that this was what I was created to do! My heart sang with praises as God worked through me to touch the hearts of many!

On May 12, 2001, ten months after I arrived in Botswana, something strange happened. I went for a jog and was praying in my mind as I ran. Out of nowhere a thought ran across my mind. "You will marry Percy Thaba." Although Francistown was his hometown, I had never met Percy because he had been away at university in Gaborone the entire ten months I had been in Botswana. His younger sister, Micky, however, was one of my most dedicated youth. She spoke often of her big brother with admiration. All the other girls spoke highly of him as well, saying he would be any girl's dream catch, but he only had eyes for God. Unbeknown to him, girls called him the holy hunk. They spoke of him like he was some saint; I always laughed to myself as I overheard them. Although I had been curious to see why this Motswana young man was so different and had captured all the girls' respect, it had never occurred to me to think of him romantically. I was there to do missions. Truly, that was my focus.

Additionally, I was born and raised in South Georgia. I had never seen a black and white couple growing up. I had only heard of them or seen it on T.V. I went to a sorority dance one time in college with a black friend I had met in one of my classes, and my mom had been really concerned over what people would think of me! No, it had never crossed my mind to consider dating anyone I met in Botswana.

Nevertheless, the thought kept coming. "You will marry Percy Thaba." I told God he had dialed the wrong number. I loved my African friends, but there was no way I was marrying an African man! I started going on with all the reasons it just would NOT work out! What would my mother say? What would our kids look like? What color would they be? What kind of hair would they have?

Then I began thinking of all the books I had read on marriage preparation. They typically recommended that couples be of a similar upbringing. I knew

15

Percy's family. They were a middle class family. So was my family. However, middle class in Africa and middle class in America were two different things! I also knew his family would not consider themselves to be Christians. My parents had me in church before I was even born. I went through all the reasons socially, economically, culturally, and racially that it would not be a good match.

As I thought through all of the reasons it wouldn't work, I kept hearing this still small voice in my mind softly saying, "This is the man I have for you." I analyzed all my reasons for resisting and realized that ultimately there was one main reason I didn't want to marry an African man. I was afraid of what people would think of me. As I thought about this, God reminded me again, "This is the man I have for you. Don't worry about what people say."

My legs were tired from jogging. Although the whole "conversation" had been in my mind, it felt like God and I had talked over the phone. I arrived at my house. I wiped the sweat off my brow and started stretching. I remembered the story where Gideon laid out the fleece to make sure he heard God correctly. I needed my own "fleece." As I cooled down, I looked up towards the sky and said "Okay, God if this is you, please prove it."

It was Saturday, and I led a youth group on Saturday afternoons. I went inside my house, took a shower, and headed off to church. After a few minutes, a taxi pulled up to the church. A young man that I had never seen got out of the cab. All the youth swarmed the guy. "Percy! Are you home for the winter?" (American seasons are opposite of Botswana's seasons so winter is June-August. Universities close during these months similar to the way universities close during the summer in the States.)

It was Percy's first weekend back after a year away at university. Just to be sure it was the "right" Percy, I grabbed one of my youth and asked, "Is that Micky's brother?"

He responded, "Oh yeah! You don't know Percy! He is such a cool guy!" I quietly slipped away to the bathroom and sighed. What was God up to? I didn't need this distraction.

Looking out the airplane window, I smiled. How far we had come since then! That September marked five years and some months we had been married! I could have never guessed this is how it would have turned out that Saturday so long ago at a youth group meeting in a small church in Francistown, Botswana.

I thought back to our relationship. The night after I had my "revelation", I called my mom and asked her, "Hypothetically speaking if I were to marry a black African man, what would you say?"

She said, "If he is a man of God, I wouldn't care about his color or nationality."

Shocked, I said "Could you put my mom on the phone?!" She laughed and said she was serious. Her lifelong prayer for my future spouse was that it be a man who feared the Lord and loved me. Hmm, one expected obstacle out of the way. Now, what about my boss? She knew I was here to do missions for a relatively short period of time. Dating was discouraged as it generally took the focus away from work. How would I convince her that this was "of God"?

My boss, unbeknown to me, had called Percy while he was still at school and asked him if he would partner with me that winter on his break in helping the young boys of the youth group grow in their faith. The Sunday after he arrived, she introduced us and asked me to brief Percy on our discipleship methods and start working with him. After about two weeks of working together, he shyly asked me if I could pull the car over after we had dropped off one of the boys. He told me that his feelings were starting to grow towards me and were becoming a distraction to him. He said he had made a pledge when he had become a Christian seven years earlier that he wouldn't date a girl until it was the one he would marry. Since he figured I wasn't his future wife, he had decided that the best biblical solution to his "problem" was to flee temptation. He had planned on telling me that he wasn't going to work closely with me anymore. I let him share his feelings and then told him of my run two weeks earlier and what God had revealed to me. "But", he blurted out with shock, "You are an American! It would never work!"

I replied, "I know! I told God that!"

As the year went on, God proved over and over in miraculous ways that this relationship was indeed His plan. After our initial talk, we both felt that this marriage was "arranged" by God, but we didn't love each other. We barely knew each other as most of our time getting to know each other had been simply observing the other in ministry. Apart from our revealing conversation, we had never spent time alone talking. Through some God ordained events, we became well acquainted over his winter break during various ministry opportunities we were asked to do together. When he went back to school in September, I realized I really did care for him. It surprised me how much I missed him. By October, I was getting afraid. I was leaving Botswana in July, headed back to the States. My two year term would be up. Percy would stay in Africa, and I would be in America. How was this going to work? If this relationship really wasn't of God, I didn't want to get my heart broken. I wanted out. I asked God once again if he would be so merciful as to give me another convincing sign.

Two weeks later, in November, Percy called me. The government of Botswana had just contacted him and told him that his grades qualified him to study abroad. They wanted to pay him to go to America and study there for four years. They would cover all his expenses. He would leave that August. His leave date was scheduled two weeks after my scheduled July departure date!

I literally jumped up and down there in my house!! "God", I chuckled, "you are too good!" Deep in my heart I knew for sure that someday God was going to bless the union of Percy Thaba and myself.

April 2002, the Botswana government issued a statement that due to some drug and alcohol problems with their stateside students, they were transferring their students from America to Canada. I was a bit concerned at the transfer, but I knew that God would somehow work it out for us to be together so I didn't worry too much. I consoled myself, thinking, at least we would be on the same continent!

After my two years in Botswana, the I.M.B. asked me to travel in America for six months, speaking to different churches and groups of college students as a mission mobilizer. I found myself again looking at my life in disbelief. What did I do to become so blessed that God would use me to encourage others to go on the mission field?

I was given a couple of weeks to spend quality time with my family and friends, whom I had left two years earlier to move to Africa. In August, I started my new job. My first assignment was to speak about the ministry opportunities in Southern Africa at a huge student conference in Glorietta, New Mexico. Along with other mission mobilizers, we were asked to set up booths for the students to be able to visually see the opportunities and ask us questions. As I looked around, I saw a booth displaying Canadian mission opportunities.

While looking at their posters, a man approached me about Canadian missions. I responded that I honestly had never thought about missions in Canada, but I was interested in being near Percy. I explained my past ministries, and he seemed to get really excited. He informed me that one of his trip goals was to locate someone to start a church specifically tailored to reach out to the 100,000 college students in Ottawa, Canada.

That same weekend in Ottawa, Canada, Percy attended a Southern Baptist church. The pastor announced that the church should pray for a man who had gone down to the States to look for someone to help start a daughter church plant geared to the thousands of college students in their city. As he explained more, Percy decided I would be perfect for the job. He approached the pastor about me after the service.

On Monday, the same man I met and Percy's pastor reported back to one another. They both said they had found a potential person for the job. When they said the name, my name, they were stunned. God had led them to the same person thousands of miles apart in different countries. They knew it was a God thing. The pastor called me, insisting they wanted me to come.

The pastor wrote the job description with an organization called the North American Mission Board (N.A.M.B.). I applied for the job specifically written for me. I still had to go for interviews but was quickly notified I had gotten the job. The next time N.A.M.B. would send out missionaries would be January 1, 2003. My six month job with the International Mission Board finished December 31, 2002. I would finish my job and start the new one on the next day!

Everything worked out perfectly with the timing, the location, and the job. Soon I found myself living in Ottawa Canada. I got to do what I loved (missions) AND to be with the one I loved! Percy and I sat amazed at how faithful God was at taking care of all of our needs.

My new job focused on reaching out to the students at Percy's university! Are you kidding me, I thought? God you are brain cell blowing!! Only you could allow me to meet my future husband in Botswana and then give me a job at his university in Canada during his four years abroad doing what I am so passionate about! The church plant prospered, and we daily watched as students from literally all over the world turned their lives around to follow the one true God of the universe! Hallelujah!

Percy's senior year started coming to an end; we had to decide our next move. We had immensely enjoyed our Canadian experience; however, we both knew that it was a place God had called us to for a season. The question for us was whether we should return to my home in the States or to Botswana. After seeking God, He led us to my hometown of Tifton Georgia for a two year stint. We both sensed that God was calling us to Botswana for life, but we felt our marriage would be healthier if he had a better understanding of where I came from. Percy had only met my parents on three vacations and our wedding. He had only seen pictures of most of my friends and family. He had never experienced any significant amount of time in the culture and family that so greatly shaped who I was.

After the first year in the States passed, we began to prepare to go back to Botswana. Without a doubt, we knew God was calling us back to Botswana. We didn't know why, but we were confident He had a plan for us! I yearned to get back to my beloved African country and tell everyone I met about the goodness of life walking with their Creator and living by His Spirit. We applied with the International Mission Board. I had been working with the Southern Baptist for fifteen years at that point. When I thought of missions, I thought of the I.M.B. I couldn't imagine a life of missions without the support and structure of their organization.

Sadly, we quickly found out that since Percy was a "national" to Botswana, we no longer qualified to work with the *International* Mission Board. Without the support of I.M.B, the move suddenly became very scary. To go back now would mean we needed to buy a one way ticket out of our savings. We would go back with no means to support ourselves and live with his parents until we could find a job and house. On top of all that, we were dragging a nine-month-old baby girl into a foreign country. With I.M.B., they would have supported us fully and had a house waiting on us when we got to Botswana. All our medical bills would be covered; the kids' schooling would be subsidized; and should any problem ever occur that made the place dangerous in which to live, a way would be provided to get us out. Also, we would have an instant "family" there with other likeminded American missionaries to celebrate holidays and talk with on lonely days when I missed home. Another tremendous benefit to working with the I.M.B was the regular furloughs that would allow us to go back to the States for six months or longer to see my family. Going back like this meant we had no idea when we would ever see my parents again. My children would surely grow up, most likely, never knowing their wonderful maternal grandparents. Going without an organization meant I was going back simply as Percy's wife. I would have no "special" rights as a missionary. I would be going back with the heart of an American missionary but with the identity of any other African housewife. Had we really heard God?

We prayed, fasted, and sought His guidance. Clearly, God led us both to the scripture in Genesis 12:1 (NIV). *"The LORD had said to Abram, "Leave your country, your people and your father's household and go to the land I will show you."* Hey! At least we knew the land ahead of time! ☺ People commended us for our "leap of faith"; but in all honesty, there was no other option for us. We knew what God wanted us to do.

We bought the tickets, and Percy and I began packing to move our little family to Botswana. When we arrived at the airport, my parents got special permission to walk us to our gate. As we boarded the plane, I experienced something that broke my heart. It was something I had never seen before. My father began to weep. My father was not an emotional man. He generally had a straight face no matter what was happening. He rarely got upset or yelled. Likewise, he rarely laughed and got overly excited either. He was a calm, quiet man; as he hugged my daughter, his first and only grandchild at the time, goodbye, not knowing when he would ever see her again, he broke down.

I opened my eyes and looked around. The medical rescue men sat calmly watching my critically ill newborn son. The engine quietly hummed as the pilot and co-pilot softly chatted. Here I was on a plane again, but Percy wasn't sitting beside me and Anna Catherine wasn't crawling all over me. I still had fresh memories of people crying, like the last time I had left loved ones and boarded a plane. However, this time the tears were much different. This time my friends had cried as we left Botswana because they literally didn't know if they would ever see Caleb again.

Chapter Three

Arrival in a place of hope

Caleb and I arrived in Pretoria, South Africa late on Wednesday night. The hospital admitted him into the neonatal intensive care unit (N.I.C.U.). They immediately assessed him as critical, calling the doctors from their homes to come treat Caleb. When the doctors came, I could tell the nurses didn't want me to hear what they were saying as they briefed them on his condition. Their faces were serious and sad, but they were obviously trying to be kind to me. They politely ushered me into a waiting room and asked if I could just sit and wait there while they conversed. After a little while, the pediatric neurologist came in and said calmly, "Your son is in a life-threatening condition. Tonight is very critical. He is severely dehydrated so we will flush him with fluids and try and get his kidneys working again. We will also give him a strong medication to stop the seizures. We will put him on oxygen and monitor him very closely. It is a good thing you brought him here. He probably wouldn't have made it very much longer in his current state." What I heard confirmed my suspicions. If they couldn't reverse the damage done in Botswana, my son would die!

The doctor went home and I was left reeling from the news. A nurse came in and put her arm around me like a child and guided me to a small kitchen. "Have you eaten anything today?" she asked compassionately. Oh, food! I actually couldn't remember when I last ate. She made me a sandwich and sat beside me. My hands were shaking as I tried to hold a cup of hot tea she placed in my hands. At first, she just sat in silence seeming to inaudibly tell me that she was available if I wanted to talk. Then she started to speak slowly. "I am so sorry. He is so dehydrated. That is one of the simplest forms of medical care he should have received." She stopped and shook her head as if to force herself to be positive with me. "I don't know what kind of doctors were treating your son in Botswana, but I can promise you, we will do everything we can to help your son. You have come to a good place. If you have any questions, feel free to ask. We have staff working 24 hours a day. We have many nurses on staff each shift to ensure each baby receives all the attention he/she needs."

Having come from a hospital in Botswana where they had a tiny "nursery" with all the babies both healthy and sick combined together, with one nurse in charge of all feedings, diaper changes, shots, etc., I was greatly encouraged! Finally, it sounded like my son would get adequate medical treatment! Wait; there was one more concern I had. I stated, "In my research, I have read it is best to touch and talk to a baby even if he is not responsive. Will I be allowed to hold him?"

"SURE! We agree!" she assured me. "We want you to touch him as much as possible!" Oh, this was too good to be true! After coming from a place where no one would communicate with me about my son's medical conditions, his constant seizures were going basically unnoticed and definitely not attended to, where my only contact with him was sticking my hand through a small hole in a plastic box, and where my husband wasn't even allowed in the same room with his son, this news was music to my ears!

I needed to pass the time until Percy came. What was the best thing I could do? I asked the nurse if I could bother her with one small request. Could I have a piece of paper and pen? I wanted to write my prayer team. I wasn't sure when I would have internet access, but I wanted to write my thoughts down while they were "raw".

Oh, how thankful I was that the International Mission Board had required us to form a prayer team before I went on staff with them as a journeyman 10 years earlier. As ministry had taken me around the world, the prayer team had grown so large that I actually didn't even know how big it was anymore. Their replies to my emails always gave me encouragement and spurred me on in my journey with Christ. They acted as a "therapist" allowing me to vent, to share joys, to ask questions, and to praise God with them. I never felt judged even on my darkest days when I shared the ugly truth about what I was feeling that day. I always felt surrounded with love by these godly friends! Frequently, as I processed my thoughts and experiences to update them, God had spoken to me as I had written. Blessed is an understatement of how I felt to have such a support system cheering for me. I knew that at the punch of a key, I could send an email off into cyberspace and hundreds around the world would join me in my African sagas! I knew I would be lifted up to the throne of the King of Kings by these people. I knew I would be carried along on the backs of these saints who so faithfully interceded on my behalf.

As I sat there thoughts about my prayer team filled me with utmost gratitude for their part in my life! Yes, I wanted to write my prayer team!

Among other things I wrote, *"Pray for Caleb, because he is still not responsive and showing no reflexes (sucking, grasping, etc) The nurses have pricked him with countless needles and stuck cords down his nose and over his face and he hasn't moved. He hasn't cried out in pain or made any sound for that matter. Lord, if possible take this cup ----but not my will, but Your will be done. Continue to pray for us. Pray for our peace and for His grace. Obviously, we want perfect healing for Caleb. We want to be able to take our son and hold him and I want to feed him. We want Anna Catherine to know her brother. We want to comfort him and cuddle him and to hear him cry. But, Lord not my will but Your will be done."*

By the time I had finished writing, Percy had arrived. His boss had driven the five hour trip just to drop him off and then return to Botswana. I told Percy with excitement, "They are going to let you touch him here!" At that point, he was still too fragile to actually hold but at least we could have contact with him as our fingers searched for places on his body that weren't covered in the web of cords and wires providing life support to his tiny body. Percy immediately went over and laid his hands on Caleb, praying for him as he tenderly placed kisses all over his unresponsive face.

The hospital had guestrooms, two floors above N.I.C.U. that were reserved for guardians of people who were receiving long term care. Fortunately, one of the few rooms was available. We rented it for the week and fell in bed exhausted, hoping tomorrow would bring better news.

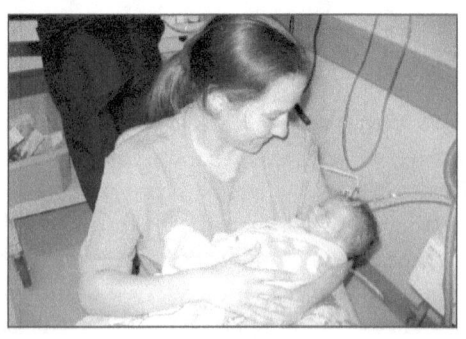

Me holding Caleb in the hospital

Chapter Four

Climbing up the mountain

Thursday morning, September 10th, brought rays of sunshine peering through the curtains into our room. Birds chirped cheerfully outside. All seemed right with the world as I woke up in the clean, crisp hospital bed sheets. I looked around and took it all in. Where was I again? So much was happening that I had to shake my groggy head and rub my eyes. It all flooded back to me. I was in a hospital in South Africa. My 4-day-old baby son laid critically ill downstairs. We had taken an emergency evacuation and flown in here last night. Did he make it through the night? I shook Percy softly and urged we check on Caleb.

We soon found ourselves at his bedside. He still lay motionless as the nurses bustled around the room from patient to patient. We summoned a lady and asked for the update on our little guy. We were informed there was a bit of improvement, but he was still critical. While we were there, a nurse beckoned us to her office. She informed us that our medical aid had called and said that they wanted to make sure we understood that our policy only covered up to 60,000 rands (about 8,000 U.S. dollars) for a hospital stay. We had been there less than 24 hours and our bill was already at 27,000 rands!! We paid 1,000 pula (the Botswana pula is a stronger currency than the Rand) a month for that insurance! "Surely there must be some mistake" I exclaimed! She said she also was surprised since their local insurance companies usually covered up to half a million rands or more. She had even called and spoken with them personally. There was nothing she could do. That was their policy.

I didn't know what to say. Percy stepped in and queried, "How long do you think we will be here?" The nurse reminded us that ultimately the doctor determines the length of his stay but based on her experience, children like

Caleb stay for months before being released. "What are our options here?" Percy probed. Basically, we could stay however long they thought best, and , agree in writing, that we would cover the rest out of our pockets or we could be transferred to a public government hospital where the care was free.

"But you should know", she looked into our eyes as if wanting to say something but knowing she shouldn't, "you get what you pay for." Catching her drift, we knew Caleb needed to stay in this hospital if we wanted him to improve.

We looked at each other, reading each other's thoughts. With a determined look on his face, Percy declared with certainty, "Our Father owns the cattle on a thousand hills. Give us the papers to sign. We will pay out of our pockets if we have to, but Caleb stays here." I poked Percy when she left the paperwork and joked "Great, now she thinks we are ranchers or farmers or something!" Later, we learned, however, she was familiar with our "cattle" Bible verse and was encouraged by our giant leap of faith.

It was scary signing a piece of paper knowing that we could very well be signing away our life savings! Our love for Caleb and our trust that God would take care of all our needs gave us strength to do what we felt we needed to do. Still, it was overwhelming.

We returned to Caleb's bedside. His head was now covered with different colored wires sticking out, bound by a bandage around his forehead. This was an EEG test, we were told, to help monitor the internal activity of his brain. They instructed us not to touch him during the testing, so I pulled out my camera to take a picture for our prayer team.

The last picture viewed filled the screen. After pressing play, Anna Catherine appeared singing and dancing in a short video taken the day before I went into labor with Caleb. Tears and smiles overwhelmed my face at the same time. For almost two years, she had constantly been at my side and somehow she had this ability to make me smile even on my worst days! I felt hollow inside. I missed our little girl. I had left her indefinitely back in Botswana. Was I a bad mother for doing that? I had just left our baby girl! At that time we didn't know the family that had taken her very well. We had only spoken with them a handful of times. But we had been desperate and they had been willing to take her. Oh how I wished I could just hug her and have something worth smiling about in my arms!

I looked up from the camera and caught Percy looking at me like he was pondering some deep thought. "What?" I questioned.

"Umm", he started hesitantly "I don't know if this is the right time but we need to talk about something important. I only took a week's leave for Caleb's birth you know. It is Thursday and I am supposed to be back at work on Monday." I didn't even let him finish before I exploded. "You have GOT to be kidding me! You are NOT leaving me in a foreign country with a sick baby while I LIVE in a hospital getting pushed from place to place by strangers because I can't even WALK due to all the physical pain I am in! NO WAY!"

Being an understanding man, he didn't snap back at me but lovingly said "I understand that this is important Ashley but we just signed a paper committing that we would pay an unknown amount of money. We can't afford to lose my job!" I understood what he meant so I couldn't respond. I just hugged him tightly and wept. The smiles were gone.

Surrounded by the sterile halls of a foreign hospital, I felt hopeless. Nurses rushed by to attend patients. Parents walked by with blood shot eyes wiping away tears. The intercom boomed out loud announcements that echoed through the corridors paging doctors to come immediately to the latest emergency. Screams of pain came from the children's ward. Nothing breathed hope and life to me. Instead, sickness and sadness suffocated me. I needed to get out of this place. I needed fresh air.

My excruciating pain (from what I later found out was a botched job on my stitches as well) prevented me from walking. Luckily, since we were in a hospital, wheelchairs were easy to find, but they couldn't leave the premises. A leisurely stroll outside was out of the question. I felt trapped. My aching head fell into my hands as I cried out to God to rescue me. God's words penetrated my bleak thoughts, turning me to His truth, that no matter where I was or what condition I was in, there was always a way out!

Some verses that came to mind were:

"*Cast all your anxiety on him because he cares for you.*" 1 Peter 5:7 (NIV)

"*⁶Do not be anxious about anything, but in everything, by prayer and petition, with thanksgiving, present your requests to God. [7]And the peace of God, which transcends all understanding, will guard your hearts and your minds in Christ Jesus."* Philippians 4:6-7 (NIV)

"God is our refuge and strength, an ever-present help in trouble. [2] Therefore we will not fear, though the earth gives way and the mountains fall into the heart of the sea..." Psalms 46:1-2(NIV)

"Let us then approach the throne of grace with confidence, so that we may receive mercy and find grace to help us in our time of need." Hebrews 4:16 (NIV)

I knew where I would find a place of refuge; it wasn't outside. "Percy," I nudged, "Let's get to the room so we can be alone." We had a date with God that we couldn't afford to miss! I knew I was literally going to fall apart without His intervention!

Up in our room, Percy helped me out of the wheelchair and eased me onto the bed. He retrieved our Bibles and sat down beside me. Now what? We knew we needed to meet with God, but how? We weren't in a church or some beautiful setting outdoors surrounded by picturesque scenery. We were in an empty hospital room filled with grief and frustration, still reeling from the shock of everything that was happening! We hadn't planned a "retreat" with God. How did we meet with God with such unprepared hearts?

I remembered reading a verse somewhere in Isaiah claiming that in repentance and rest we would find salvation. I flipped to Isaiah and found it in Isaiah 30:15. *"This is what the Sovereign LORD, the Holy One of Israel, says: "In repentance and rest is your salvation, in quietness and trust is your strength..."* We understood the "rest" part of the verse. We had both decided until we had regained some semblance of sanity, we weren't leaving the room. After all, we had nowhere to go! We were stuck in a hospital! We were sitting on the bed because our deepest desire was to find rest in God.

Now, we needed to address the repentance part of the verse. I didn't need to search my heart very long or hard before I uncovered harbored bitterness! The pediatrician and gynecologist working at the hospital in Botswana charged us a ton of money and for what -- ridiculously negligent care! An innocent baby's life now hung in jeopardy due to their carelessness—my innocent baby. And, what was worse, they were arrogant, rude, and completely apathetic towards us also! I seethed just thinking about them. Could I really honestly say I was sorry for being mad at them? Could I intentionally choose to forgive them for their actions? It was starting to look like Caleb had some major brain damage that was going to compromise his standard of life. Maybe that day I could say I had forgiven them, but in five years, if Caleb couldn't walk or talk, could I truly forgive them?

I recalled the story of Joseph in the Bible. His brothers wanted him dead. They didn't care about him. Their actions had, in every way, been evil and cruel. However, when Joseph looked back on his life he made a comment that stuck out to me. "*You intended to harm me, but God intended it for good to accomplish what is now being done, the saving of many lives.*" Genesis 50:20 (NIV). Romans 8:28 came to mind where we are reminded that all things work together for the good of those who love the Lord. I thought of Romans 13:1, which said, "*Everyone must submit himself to the governing authorities, for there is no authority except that which God has established. The authorities that exist have been established by God.*" A pattern emerged. God was telling me, through His word, that regardless if the authorities or people in our lives meant good or evil in the things they did in our lives, ultimately we were still called to trust in God. In His sovereignty, if He chose not to intervene, then somehow it would work for my good because I knew I loved the Lord!

I pondered this for awhile. As I continued to think about it, it began to free me from my bitterness. I decided that playing the blame game would do nothing to change the past or the future. It would just take my thoughts away from focusing on heaven and what its reality brought to my earthly existence. I knew God loved me. I knew God had a plan to prosper me and not to harm me. I knew God promised me an abundant life. I had an intimate relationship with my perfect heavenly Father and had learned through experience that He always took care of me. So, if God allowed this, then if anything I should be mad at God, theoretically. But there is NO way that option entered my mind! I had decided a long time ago that I agreed with Peter when Jesus asked him if he would leave when times got tough. Simon Peter answered him, "*Lord, to whom shall we go? You have the words of eternal life. We believe and know that you are the Holy One of God.*" John 6:68-69 (NIV)

I actually started getting excited as the truth sunk in. If God allowed this, then some good was going to come out of it. How could I be mad at the doctors? Somehow their harmful actions were going to bring us good. The words of John 9 came to my mind again. When Jesus was asked whose sin caused the man to be born blind, He responded that this was done so that the work of God might be displayed in that man's life. Once more, God quietly whispered that He would get glory out of Caleb's life.

Naturally, my next was question was HOW He was planning on getting the glory from Caleb's life. In the blind man's story, his parents claimed he was at a mature enough age to speak for himself. That meant the blind man got healed but not until he was older. Was God saying He would heal Caleb but it would be after everyone had seen just how bad he was so that people would know it was truly a miracle? Was God saying He would heal him instantly? Was God saying He wanted to get glory out of the situation because we chose to praise Him even if He never healed him? I needed more clarification.

Satan's conversation with God in Job's story popped into my mind, *"Does Job fear God for nothing?" Satan replied. "Have you not put a hedge around him and his household and everything he has? You have blessed the work of his hands, so that his flocks and herds are spread throughout the land. But stretch out your hand and strike everything he has, and he will surely curse you to your face."* Job 1:9-11 (NIV)

God had blessed me in my life! There was no doubt about that! On more than one occasion when I had shared the gospel with someone, they had replied critically, "Of course, you can believe in God. Nothing seriously bad has ever happened to you. You have no reason to doubt His existence." What if I prayed tirelessly for Caleb, and he still couldn't walk or talk. Yet, I still chose to willingly proclaim God's goodness and power. Surely people would know that I truly loved the Lord.

I thought of the story of Shadrach, Meshach, and Abednego. They were told to bow down to a foreign god or get thrown in a fiery furnace. They chose the furnace. Before they were thrown in, the king taunted them, saying that no god could rescue them now. They responded with conviction that their God COULD save them from the fire but EVEN IF HE DIDN'T, they would NOT bow to another god. I knew God COULD heal Caleb, but I decided EVEN IF HE DIDN'T, I would not turn my back on him.

I thought of Paul in the Bible. Paul gave his entire life to spreading the message of God's redemptive plan throughout the world in his day. If anyone deserved to be blessed in every way, it was Paul. Yet 2 Corinthians 11:24-27 records Paul saying the following. *"²⁴Five times I received from the Jews the forty lashes minus one. ²⁵Three times I was beaten with rods, once I was stoned, three times I was shipwrecked, I spent a night and a day in the open sea, ²⁶I have been constantly on the move. I have been in danger from rivers, in danger from bandits, in danger from my own countrymen, in danger from Gentiles; in danger in the city, in danger in the country, in danger at sea; and in danger from false brothers. ²⁷I have labored and toiled and have often gone without sleep; I have known hunger and thirst and have often gone without food; I have been cold and naked."* In Philippians 4:11-13, Paul says ... *"I have learned to be content whatever the circumstances. ¹²I know what it is to be in need and I know what it is to have plenty. I have learned the secret of being content in any and every situation, whether well fed or hungry, whether living in plenty or in want. ¹³I can do everything through Him who gives me strength."*

In reading the accounts of Paul's life, I realized that Paul came to understand that an abundant life had nothing to do with external circumstances. An abundant life meant no matter what my circumstances were, with Christ's strength, I could do anything. With His Spirit, although externally I may waste away, inwardly I was going to be renewed day by day. If I remained in Christ, I would be full of love, joy, peace, patience, kindness, goodness, faithfulness, gentleness, and self control. And, no matter what happened, I could be confident that this life was but a breath, and ultimately, I would spend eternity in a place where there would be no more death or pain.

The last example I thought about was my Savior himself. On the eve His painful crucifixion, the Bible records that He was full of sorrow to the point of death. He wished there was another way but in the end He said that He didn't want his will but wanted to do God's will. Not only me, but millions around the world for centuries have benefitted from His selfless decision. I was so thankful that He didn't follow his desires but trusted in God. God's ways sometimes didn't make sense at the time, but in hindsight, every person who walked in obedience always had reason to praise God when the time of trouble had passed.

I believed that something good was going to come out of this situation, but even if it wasn't exactly what I prayed for, it wouldn't change God's identity. He was still the Alpha and the Omega! He was still the Creator of all six billion people that inhabit planet earth. He still spoke light into darkness and held the keys to eternity. He still was the most powerful force in the universe. He still sent His son to die for me, and He still remained my best friend. Right then, no matter what happened, I decided God would always be worthy of my worship and hold the place of Master in my life. He had no match, for truly there was none like Him. I announced confidently to Percy, "No matter what happens, I will choose to praise God!"

My off key voice joined with Percy's beautiful voice as we sang joyfully to the Lord. We passionately sang songs like "I surrender all" as we pondered the unknown road ahead. Song after song spilled from our hearts. I didn't know what God's will was for Caleb or what his future held. I did, however, know God's will for me. He had clearly outlined that in 1 Thessalonians 5: 16-18 where I am instructed to "*be joyful always; pray continually; give thanks in all circumstances, for this is God's will for you in Christ Jesus.*" As we continued to praise Him, the fruit of the Spirit flowed naturally! We were not trying to be joyful. His spirit just led us to feel that emotion. We were not trying to be peaceful. We had just given this over to God and were filled with a peace which surpassed understanding and guarded our hearts and minds in Christ Jesus. I was on my knees, but I felt like I was touching the heavens!

After about an hour, we were ready to leave our sanctuary. There had been a few times in my life where I could say I was on a spiritual high. That day I felt like I climbed to the mountaintop with God. He had ministered to me in His courts. Some people get to experience God on beautiful weekend retreats in exotic lands. I guess God knew I needed something more drastic. He brought me to the bedside of my brain damaged first born son to lead me to a place of complete peace and intimacy with him.

We returned to the N.I.C.U. Outwardly, I looked the same with my stringy unwashed hair and puffy red eyes. Since I had been confined to the hospital on the morning of our evacuation, Percy had packed my bags. He had packed clothes I commonly used, not thinking that after the birth, those clothes would fall off me. Only two outfits actually fit my post-pregnancy body. Therefore, I was daily forced to wear the same dirty clothes even though dried milk stains covered the front of both shirts because I had no baby to feed, but my milk had come in nonetheless. Contrary to my unchanged disheveled outward appearance, inwardly, I was a different person! I had met with God!

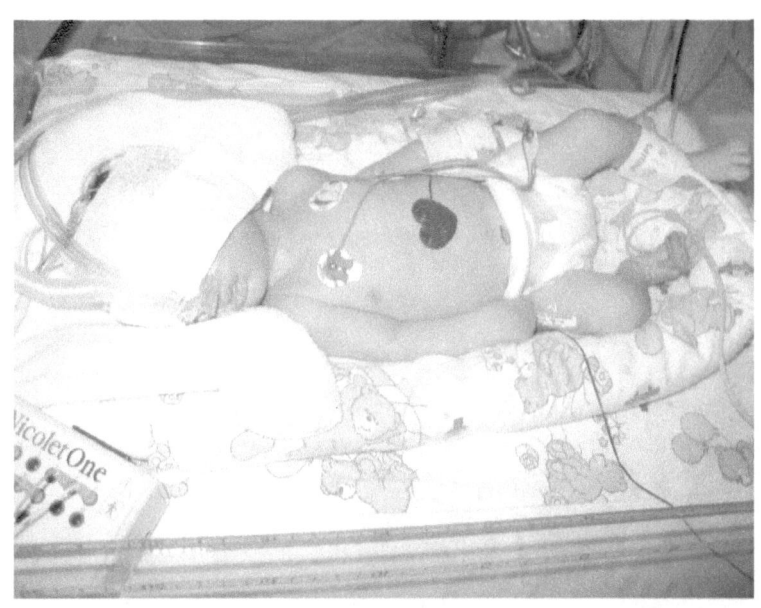

Caleb on his bed in the N.I.C.U. in South Africa

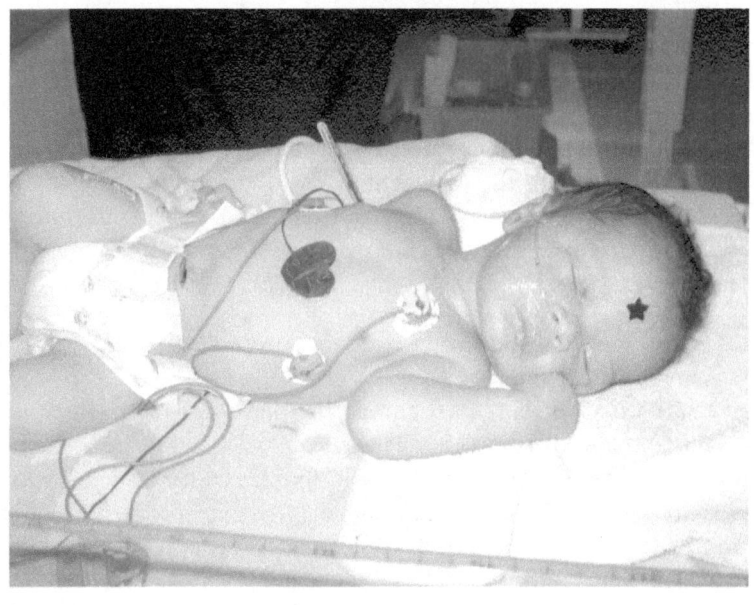

Chapter Five

Doom's day

The peace of God continued to reign in our hearts as we woke up on Friday, September 11, 2009. We hurried downstairs to visit Caleb and check his progress. The nurses informed us that since we had gone to bed last night he had only had five obvious seizures. The EEG had shown a few more internal ones that weren't apparent outwardly. He still wasn't healthy, but it showed he was responding to the medicine and the seizures were decreasing.

They also reported that he had started taking my breast milk. Since birth, he had been on a drip with a watery solution being deposited directly into his arm. He still didn't have the ability to swallow on his own, but they wanted to try him on the heavier, more nutrient dense breast milk. Therefore, they put a tube down his nose straight to the stomach. He held down the first 5 ml. but couldn't keep down the 10 ml, attempted at the next feeding. They reverted to 5 ml. again, slowly increasing the amount at each three hour feeding. By the time we arrived that morning, he was taking 20 ml. of my milk through the tube. The rest of his fluid intake was still given intravenously.

All in all, they were impressed with his improvement. Since he was becoming more stable, they thought it was safe to unhook him from all his machines for the thirty minutes it would take to do an M.R.I. brain scan. In order to transport him downstairs to the lab, they needed to move him from his bed to a portable cot. They took all his wires off and asked Percy to hold him while they set everything back up on a little portable stretcher. Percy rejoiced in the precious gift of a few minutes to cradle our son close to his body like any normal baby. Caleb was five days old, and it was only the second time Percy had held Caleb. And he had done it without Caleb being attached to numerous machines. We smiled at each other over the little blanketed bundle in his arms. Then, the moment was over as someone gently took Caleb. They told us sometime that afternoon they would give us the reports of the EEG and the M.R.I., and they wheeled our son away.

At breakfast, some friends surprised us with a visit holding a most coveted laptop with internet access. They knew I urgently wanted to send an email to my prayer team. We chatted for a bit, but within a couple of minutes, I couldn't contain my excitement any longer. I excused myself and scurried off to write my needed prayer letter.

With a smile on my face and a twinkle in my eye, I began pounding away on the keyboard, sharing of our glorious meeting with God the day before and the awesome lessons He had taught us. In summary, I shared how we had decided to surrender all and accept whatever fate God had for us. The tone of the email was upbeat and joyful. Halfway through the email, the nurse came into the maternity ward guest room and informed us that the doctor was ready to report his findings. I saved my work, and we followed them into the N.I.C.U. Our friends assured us that they would be right there waiting to hear the news.

When we turned the corner, my heart fluttered. Most of the nurses were gathered there with the doctor. Why were there so many of them, and why did it look like they had been crying? Some were still sniffling. The pediatric neurologist put the first scan up on the board and turned on a light behind it so we could see it clearly. He pointed to a white spot and told us that was a patch that had been damaged by lack of oxygen. The whole brain was covered in white patches and streaks! "So", I asked in shock, "All of those white areas are hurt?! That is the whole brain!" He sadly nodded yes confirming the horrifically, widespread injuries to Caleb's brain. He began pointing out specific areas of concentrated damage. I drew out my notepad and fervently took notes.

I wrote as fast as I could, trying to keep up with him as he talked. The right frontal lobe had a large hematoma that would most likely cause him to lose the function of that part of the brain. There was a bad subdural bleed that extended over the cerebellum and around the occipital lobe. There was bleeding in the pituitary gland and in the back on the neck. There was… I couldn't keep up anymore. The bleeding was too much; the damage was too extensive. I dropped the pen and began to weep. I think there was more he could have said, but he realized we had heard enough for that day and stopped reviewing the scans.

Everyone was silent. I glanced up and saw a tear drop down Percy's face. I surveyed the room full of faces. They were also full of despair and sympathy. I took a deep breath and faced the doctor. "What caused this?" He looked into my eyes, as if asking himself if I could handle the truth. Then, he slowly stated that this was caused by Caleb's traumatic delivery. He said that when they saw the labor was not progressing, they should have done a caesarean. The force of the forceps most likely caused the terrible internal bleeding. He could tell by the age of the blood that all of this damage had happened on Monday during his birth. He went on to say that *I had gone into labor with a completely healthy baby boy, but because of a doctor's mistake, his life was now changed forever.* This had been totally preventable! I thought back to how my gynecologist had been in a hurry to get back to the office and had just quickly snatched Caleb from my womb. I broke down again and heaved sobs. This time some of the nurses came and put their arms around me.

He asked me if I had any more questions. I shook my head, and he politely patted me on the back and walked away. I was sure after I had time to digest the news I would have plenty of questions. For now, however, I just wanted to mourn. I thought about the date, ironically, September 11th. I knew many around the world were mourning the dreadful terrorist events that happened eight years earlier on that same day. I now joined them. I had different reasons, but our tears were the same. We grieved over how our lives had been tragically affected by the selfish actions of others.

Percy escorted me out of the room and into the maternity ward guest room. A couple of nurses followed to make sure we were okay, asking if there was anything they could do. When we entered, our friends, who were still waiting, looked up. Their faces showed anticipation and curiosity, but they respectfully kept quiet until we were ready to relay the news. I couldn't talk. Percy shared the diagnosis while I sat with my face cradled in my hands bawling.

Later my friend asked if I wanted to finish my prayer letter. I nodded knowing our family needed prayer. I took the computer and reread what I had written before the results. The tone was so cheerful. It was hard to even remember feeling that way since I was so overwhelmed with sorrow. Heavily, I continued writing the letter. After reporting recent events, I wrote the following:

I now sit in South Africa in a hospital four days after the birth of my son knowing that I went into labor with a healthy baby boy. I am devastated to hear that it was completely preventable, and my child will never be normal short of a miracle.

I honestly don't know what else to say at this point. The doctor said there is no way we are going home before another two weeks... probably longer. That leaves Anna Catherine in Botswana, that leaves Percy having to go back to work and leaves me here (they want my breast milk and my touch on him). That leaves insane hospital bills. That leaves me sitting here powerless with nothing to do but give him my breast milk, touch him, and pray over him. I just feel so helpless. My son is lying there, and I can't do a thing to comfort him. As I said earlier, I can't even hold him most of the time and I am still in so much physical pain from the forceps delivery, the stitches and everything else, I can't even stand there by his bed for long. This is hard.

Please pray for us. I still trust the Lord. I still submit to Him. I believe his grace is sufficient for us. I know his mercies are good, and he will renew us every morning and give us the strength to get through today. I KNOW that.... but it doesn't stop the tears from falling.

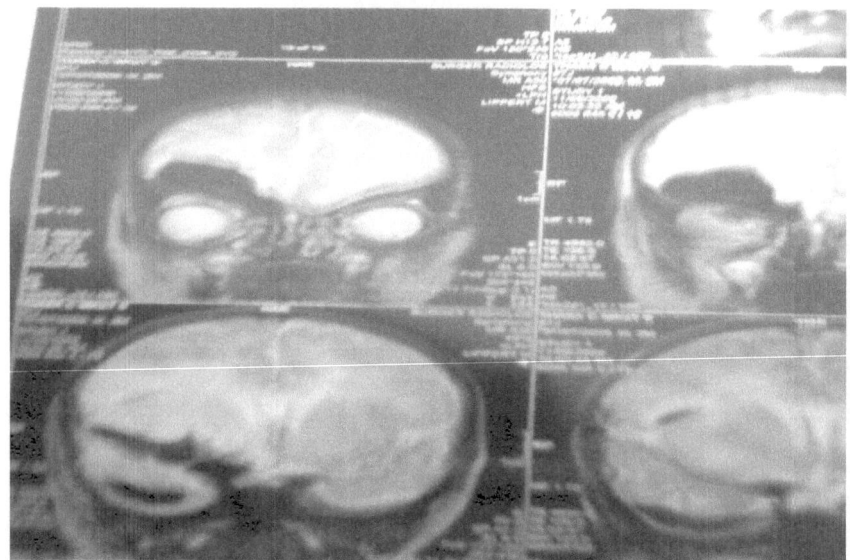

Marks correspond where the forceps squeezed his head. The skin beside his eye and on the back of his neck was broken and bleeding after birth causing ugly bruised contusions that I could see even without the scans. The scans showed how bad the damage was on the inside.

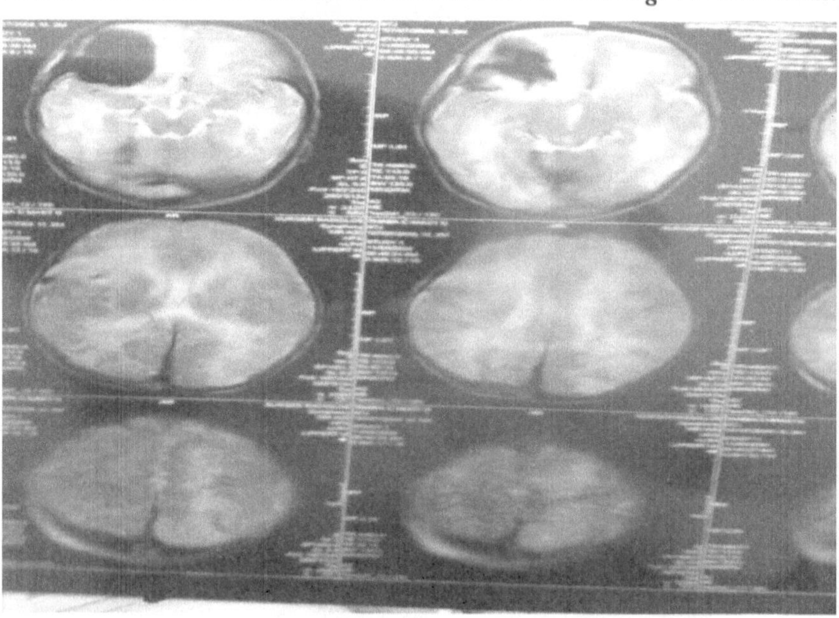

Right frontal lobe is gone and occipital lobe (bottom left) is damaged as well

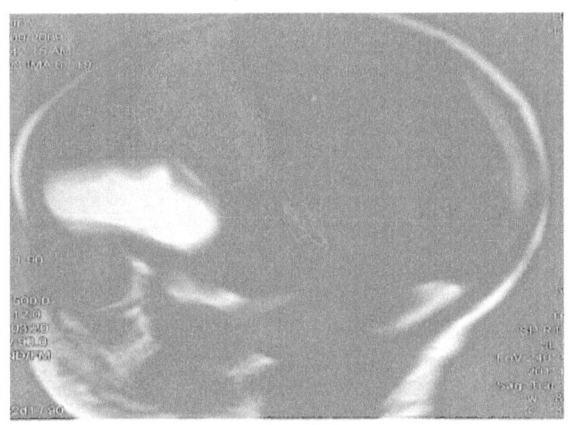

Side view showing the destroyed right frontal lobe.

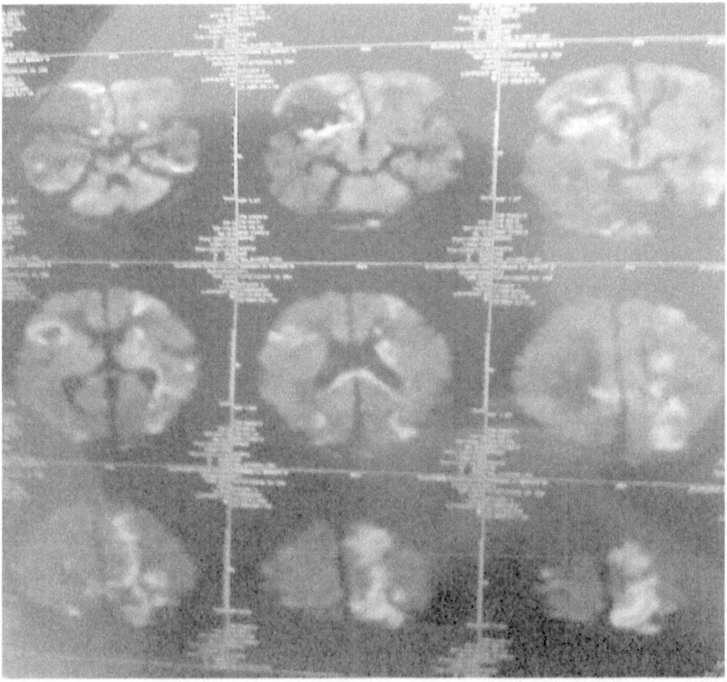

White spots show areas of damage caused by lack of oxygen. Note the concentrated damaged streak in the left hemisphere.

Chapter Six

Passing through the valley of Baca

After Percy explained the seriousness of the situation to his boss, he graciously told Percy to take as much time as he needed so that he could be there to support me. Thankfully, he was able to be with me throughout our time in the hospital. As the days turned into a week, we began to settle into a routine. We lived in the hospital. We learned the fastest route between our room and N.I.C.U, depending on what time of day it was. From the guards to the nurses, we began to greet them each by name and with a smile each day. We ordered off the room service menu. At first, the three different meal options for each meal time were appealing. However, daily eating the same food in hospital sized portions while sitting in a waiting room with a tray on our laps got old fast. Nevertheless, we memorized the menu and began to gravitate towards favorites. I liked the granola and fruit for breakfast, chicken and potatoes for lunch, and pasta primavera for dinner. It sounded better than it tasted! ☺

Talk around Caleb's bed began to move toward other subjects. We learned of each nurse's family life, kids' names, and even their religious beliefs. We decided if God had us here that we would strive to be a light in even that dark place with so much pain.

Caleb continued to improve. His kidneys were now fully functioning, though the shut down had caused a disturbing build up of calcium in the kidneys. He began showing signs of jaundice, but the nurses didn't seem worried and promised that was easy to treat.

The seizures decreased, and they began weaning him off the strong seizure medication. Although it was good news that the seizures were stopping, they were still uneasy about the damage the seizures had done. Every time he had a seizure, his oxygen level dropped. In Botswana, they pushed a tube into his incubator that constantly blew oxygen at a steady rate towards his face. In South Africa, Caleb wore a device on his foot that monitored the amount of oxygen saturation in his blood at any given moment. If at any time the oxygen levels went higher or lower than the safe standard, an alarm sounded. A nurse then came over and adjusted his oxygen amounts until he stabilized again. Therefore, contrary to the care in South Africa where his oxygen was monitored, in Botswana it always stayed at a steady rate. Subsequently, the frequent seizures he had there had caused tissue damage throughout his body and brain. There was nothing they could do about that now.

As the week wore on, his condition stabilized to the point that they were able to take off his oxygen mask and let him breathe in room air with no negative reactions. He still wore an oxygen saturation monitor on his foot, but the alarm rarely went off any more signaling dangerous saturation levels. One thing that was still a big concern was that he received all his milk through a tube. Caleb wasn't going to be released until we could feed him without the help of all the hospital machines, so we were desperate to figure out a way to get him to eat on his own. He seemed to lack either the instinct or the strength to suck. One day as we sat there, I saw some silicon bottle nipples lying on the nurse's table. It gave me an idea. I sterilized one and put cotton wool inside it so Caleb wouldn't suck in air. I began to push and pull the nipple in his mouth, mimicking the sucking motion. Percy and I alternated this exercise all day. The next day a small but very significant thing happened. My hand grew tired and I stopped for a minute, but the nipple moved ever so slightly through my fingers. "Percy, did you see that!??!" I exclaimed. He had sucked on his own! We made sure he did it a few more times on his own and then summoned a nurse with delight written all over our faces. We were proud parents with something to smile about! Our son had sucked a pacifier, even if it was just for a few seconds.

She warned us not to get too excited but promised at his next feeding she would attempt the bottle again for a small amount of his required dose of milk. After six days of either being fed through a tube inserted in his nose or intravenously, he began slowly taking milk through a bottle. At first, we celebrated because he sucked 5 ml. The rest of his needed nutrition still went through his tube straight to his stomach. Slowly, as the days passed by, he was able to suck 10 ml. and not gag or vomit. He needed to get to the standard of a normal baby who drinks, on average, 600 ml. of milk a day at that age and that weight; 600 ml. seemed so far away from 10 ml! Slowly but surely, he made it to the target 600ml. By the end of our second week, they took out the tube and relied exclusively on bottle feeding him.

I still, however, could not breastfeed. No matter how hard I tried, he just didn't have the strength to receive his milk straight from me; but it was my milk that I pumped six times daily that they fed him through the tube and later through the bottle. N.I.C.U. had strict sanitary rules, so they do not allow breast milk to sit in the refrigerator longer than a day. Each day I would pump around 1,200 ml. of breast milk or more. For days, they dumped about 1,100 ml. or more of that. I was optimistic that one day I would be able to feed my son directly. Therefore, as discouraging as it was to go through all that hard work only to literally pour it down the drain, I kept expressing, so my body would keep producing the nutrient rich milk that I knew could aid in his healing.

Since we had come, the doctor had told us that the part in his brain that regulated his body temperature must have been affected because he was either sweating profusely or cold to the touch. To help him stay at a steady temperature, they took off his clothes and left him in a diaper and paper sunglasses and put him under a hot lamp. The hot lamp was connected to a sensor placed on his chest. When his temperature dropped, it sent a message to the lamp to increase the temperature. If the temperature went up, the heat from the lamp decreased. If the landscape would have been different, he could have passed for a cool boy chilling on a sunny beach!

By the end of that second week, we had a new problem. He no longer needed the hot lamp to regulate his temperature and could lie comfortably on his bed in a footed onesie. The problem, however, was that Caleb was a full-term baby whose body was perfectly mature. The clothes they had in N.I.C.U. were mainly for premature babies. Caleb was a giant there, at his 7.7 lb.(3.5kg.) self! Since we were confined to the hospital, a thoughtful nurse shared our dilemma with a church friend. This friend graciously allowed us to borrow a bag of her son's hand me down clothes during our hospital stay. That same lady observed that Percy and I wore the same clothes every time she was at the hospital. She volunteered to launder our filthy clothes! God took care of our every need!

Our heavenly Father even granted some of our dreams as well! Our friend, Dana, who was babysitting Anna Catherine, made the five hour trek across the border just to bring our baby girl to us! The visit was surreal! She was a burst of sunshine and normalcy in our upside down world. She flitted around, blurting out story after story of all the fun things she was doing at "Aunt" Dana's house. It was obvious that she was having no problem adjusting to staying with another family and was having the time of her life! Sadly, the day quickly came to an end. As they prepared to leave, she bounced into my arms, hugging me tightly as she looked into my eyes and said "Bye Bye mommy! I love you!" Although it was hard to say goodbye for the second time in a month to my darling little girl, her vibrancy had lit up our world and gave us things to smile about for days afterwards.

Throughout the whole week, God's joy and peace was ever present in our lives. We felt very blessed to feel His Spirit so tangibly walking beside and within us. We may have been living in a hospital but we were dwelling in His courts! There is a verse we found that described how we felt. Psalms 84:4-7(NIV) states, *"Blessed are those who dwell in your house; they are ever praising you. ⁵ Blessed are those whose strength is in you, who have set their hearts on pilgrimage. ⁶ As they pass through the Valley of Baca, they make it a place of springs; the autumn rains also cover it with pools. ⁷ They go from strength to strength, till each appears before God in Zion."*

I remembered hearing a sermon one time explaining that the Valley of Baca was a place of bitterness. As the verse promised, we were passing through a difficult valley, but as we set our hearts on God, His strength allowed us to make this hard time a place where we could actually draw water and feel refreshed!

We had no idea what the future held, but we knew we could face tomorrow because He lived in us! Whenever the fears crept in, we immediately took the thoughts captive and made them obedient to Christ. When I witnessed a child being released from the hospital still with obvious disabilities, I would imagine Caleb in an even worse state and get scared. I would then remind myself of the truth that no matter what happened, God would give us the strength to get through it and somehow He would get glory out of it. I chose to surrender to His will, and moment by moment, it freed me to soar with overwhelming gratitude for how good God was!

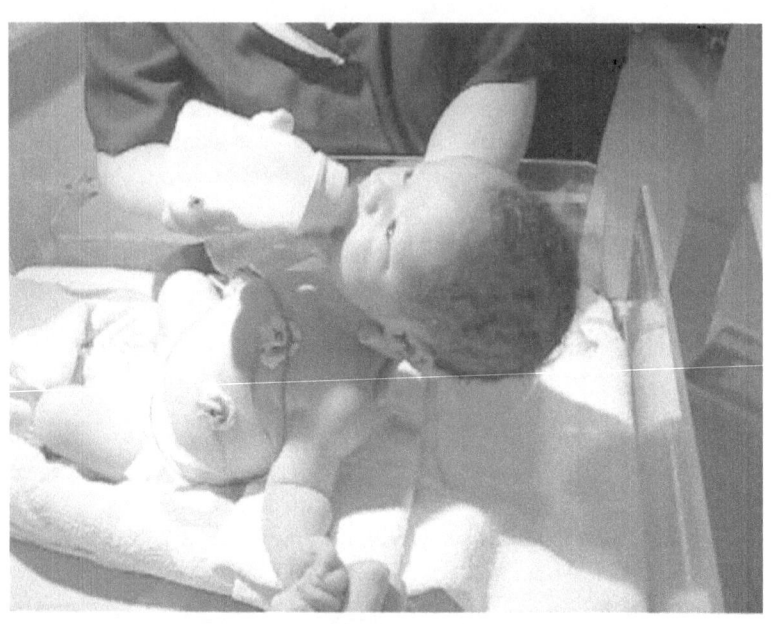

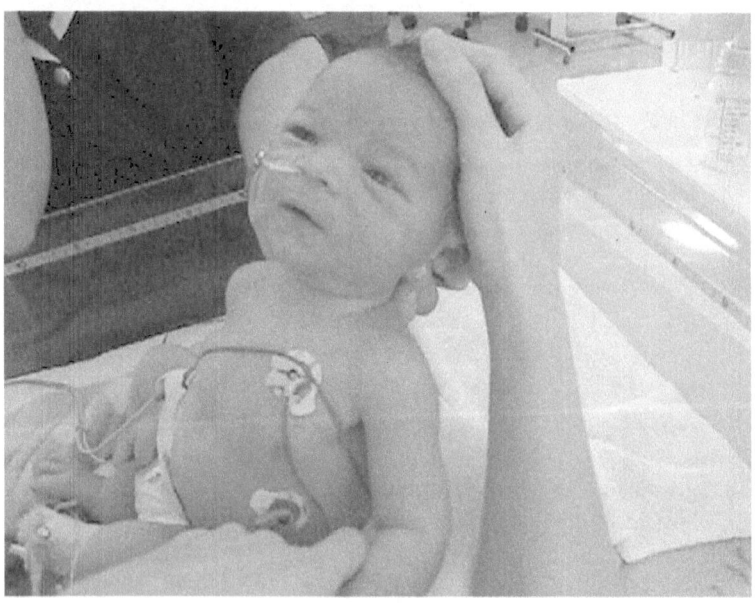

Chapter Seven

Divine intervention

Generally, we could be found in one of three places: firstly, by Caleb's bedside, talking to him, touching him, or singing and praying over him, secondly, in the maternity ward where we received our meals and I soaked my own wounds in salt water three times a day, or lastly, in our rented room. For the most part, if we weren't talking to nurses, getting updates, or discussing with each other the latest news, we were reading our Bibles in one of these three places. We were like two people who had been stuck in the desert for days without water. We felt like we needed to gulp God's words! We were so thirsty and couldn't get enough of His words to quench our souls! As we lost ourselves in seeking Him first, we felt supernaturally carried along by His strength. We were amazed at how we felt His presence so intimately!

One day during that second week, as I was sitting on our bed in our rented room, God spoke to me. The clouds didn't part nor did the sky light up with a flashing message. It was a still, small voice that interrupted my thoughts, but clearly, it was God.

I was reading the Bible when out of the blue, I thought of the story of Abraham and his son Isaac. I flipped back to Genesis and began reading the story of when he was asked by God to take his son and sacrifice him. The story wasn't new to me; I had read it more times than I could count. But, today there was something in between the written words that spoke to me. God saw that Abraham was willing to surrender his son due to his trust in God. I felt like God also saw my surrendering heart. I had truly come to a place where I was willing to say, "I trust you no matter what happens with my only son." Like Abraham, I felt God telling me, "Enough, I am giving back your son". As I prayed over what that meant, another verse came to mind. It was the story when a lady comes to Jesus and touches his garment and is healed from a bleeding disorder that had tormented her for years. In my mind, I could see that lady being healed. Then, the picture changed on my mind's wall, and I could visualize Jesus reaching down His hand and touching Caleb's head. Just as that lady's blood had dried up, I could picture the blood on Caleb's brain that had caused so much damage drying up and his brain healing.

I couldn't contain my excitement! I wanted to jump up and down and shout at the top of my lungs! God was going to heal Caleb! Percy looked over at me suspiciously and queried, "What is going on over there?"

I gushed, "God is going to heal Caleb!!!"

His face beamed with uncontainable happiness as he exclaimed, "I feel like God is telling me the same thing!" We hugged as tears of joy streamed down my face! I couldn't stop saying thank you God, thank you God, thank you God. It was crazy actually. Circumstances were the same. Nothing had changed. We had no logical reason to believe Caleb would be healed. Yet, we couldn't wipe the smiles off our faces! It was as if a doctor had knocked on our door and said, "You won't believe this. Your son is completely healed". Words really can't describe our elated states that day!

After we celebrated a bit more, we dove right back into the scriptures. We felt drawn to read about others' stories of healing throughout the Bible.

Story after story kept confirming what God had said to us. We read countless accounts of Jesus healing people. A pattern emerged that all who came to him asking in faith for healing were healed. Exodus 15:26 stated that our Father, God, is the One who heals us. Hebrews 13:8 reminded us that He is the same yesterday, today, and forever. The truth began to sink in. We served the same God of the Old Testament, and the same Jesus that healed all who came to him now lived in us. Surely, as Isaiah 59:1 stated, the arm of the LORD was not too short to save, nor his ear too dull to hear. Scripture was confirming that God indeed could and would heal Caleb.

We meditated on verses like:

When the sun was setting, the people brought to Jesus all who had various kinds of sickness, and laying His hands on each one, He healed them. Luke 4:40

Surely He took up our infirmities and carried our sorrows, yet we considered Him stricken by God, smitten by Him, and afflicted. But He was pierced for our transgressions, He was crushed for our iniquities; the punishment that brought us peace was upon him, and by His wounds we are healed. Isaiah 53:4-5

Therefore I tell you, whatever you ask for in prayer, believe that you have received it, and it will be yours. Mark 11:24

Praise the LORD, O my soul, and forget not all His benefits- who forgives all your sins and heals all your diseases. Psalms 103:2-3

Finally, we spent some time studying a story we could relate to. A man brought his sick son to Jesus and said if you can help us, take pity on us. *"If you can'?" said Jesus. "Everything is possible for him who believes."* Mark 9:23

Later that day my father called us from the States. I was practically giddy as I assured him I had good news. Naturally, when he heard the excitement in my voice, he expected us to have positive news from the doctor. I told him we had heard from a doctor alright, but it wasn't a doctor in Pretoria. We had heard from the Great Physician. After telling my dad what had happened, we asked him to join in our desire to live by faith and not by sight and change his prayers to prayers of thankfulness for God's healing. He then wrote the following email to my prayer team:

Dearly Beloved,

Your outpouring of Love has been phenomenal. Your care and concern has been outstanding. Your passionate and fervent prayers are powerful.

My prayers have run in many directions along with my emotions. But each prayer has been that I would be in obedience to the will of the Father and acknowledging that He is and always will be the only true power in the Universe. I have long since burned all bridges that lead anywhere except to Jesus as my Lord and Savior.

The faith of Ashley and Percy is the cornerstone of their lives. They too will accept God's will whatever that may be. However, today, separately they believe God told them to pray for Caleb's healing without any doubt. Ashley has asked me to ask you to do the same thing. We want you to be very specific. Believe that the God who created Caleb will heal him according to God's promises. Ask in Jesus' name that when the MRI of Caleb's brain is taken this Friday that all the blood that has caused damage will be gone, that the spasms will have stopped completely and that the damaged areas will have been restored completely. The hospital staff has said this is one of the worst cases they have seen. We pray that they will now have to admit that God had to have performed a miracle.

"And the prayer offered in faith will make the sick person well; the Lord will raise him up." James 5:15.

To God be the glory, AMEN,

Lynn Kelley

We knew the doctor wanted to do a follow up M.R.I. on Friday. We were so sure we had heard God's voice saying He had healed Caleb that we knew this time was going to be different. I could just picture the nurses and doctor looking at it in awe. I couldn't wait to show my friends and family the "before and after" shots comparing last week's scans and this week's scans. I couldn't wait to see the miracle! I couldn't wait for God to get the glory! God had revealed His power to Percy and me. Now, He was going to reveal it to all the medical staff in Unitas hospital!

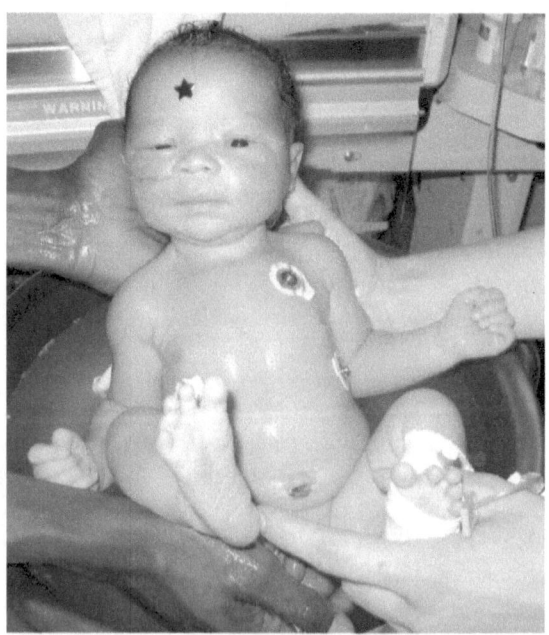

Caleb getting a bath in N.I.C.U.

Chapter Eight

An Early Release?

Things were looking up. We were expecting a good M.R.I. report. We were also expecting a long overdue visit from my parents. Oddly enough, although I was eager to see my parents, thoughts of their visit troubled me. Let me explain my heart. Since the gynecologist had pinned down Caleb's due date seven months earlier, they booked a flight and scheduled a visit to see us and meet our newborn son. It had been over a year since I last saw them. I wanted so much for this to be the perfect vacation for my parents, sharing our home, family, and country with them.

Anna Catherine was nine-months-old when we left the United States. In the past year, her personality had blossomed along with her motor and verbal skills. For months I had been watching little things she would do and imagine watching my parent's reaction when they saw her. She would run over and grab the cell phone and start jabbering to some pretend person on the other end. I could almost picture my parents cracking up with giggles watching her cute actions. I couldn't wait to "share" her with them!

Percy and I had bought a house in Botswana. Before this, I had always rented places. I had cleaned every nook and cranny so I could proudly show our first home off to my parents, especially my mom. I excitedly reorganized and spruced up Anna Catherine's room in anticipation of their visit, even purchasing a new bed and sheets so they wouldn't have to sleep on an air mattress beside her crib. This was going to be a special time!

I had never been "great" in the kitchen and had rarely cooked for myself before I married Percy. It concerned my mom and she frequently made comments about my bad eating habits and my need to become more domesticated. However, a husband and a child changed all that. I wouldn't claim to be a gourmet chef, but I had certainly learned how to cook up a few delicious meals. For months, after a meal Percy, would say, "Oh, that one was really good. Put it on the list to make for your mom." It became the house joke. No, that meal wasn't "mother worthy" or that one definitely made the cut! I kept records and made a list of meals I wanted to make sure I cooked for her. I was happy about the new "me" I was going to share with my mom.

With Percy consumed with work and me being so busy at home with Anna Catherine, I was clueless as to what kinds of fun things Gaborone had to offer. We rarely travelled further than the grocery store. Definitely, there was no time to explore the prized local tourist attractions. I determined, though, to uncover the gems of our city, seeking out answers from all our more socially active friends. Yes, a newborn would curtail our outings, but this was going to be a memorable time for Mom and Dad nonetheless.

Those dreams washed away the day Caleb was born. Our world needed to revolve around him. Consequently, we were stuck in a hospital. Anna Catherine was miles away. Only parents were allowed into N.I.C.U. so we didn't even know if they would get to touch Caleb. There would be no playing with Anna Catherine, no cuddling their new grandson, no experiencing our wonderful Gaborone, and no sleeping in our new bed. I knew I had bigger issues, but this also made me sad. They were coming for three weeks, and now this whole ordeal was going to cost me my dream holiday with them!

Percy understood my frustration, but he gently encouraged me to make the best out of the situation. He was right. I tried busying myself changing their flight, so they could join us in Pretoria and booking a guest house near the hospital. I even tried to plan a few day trips to nearby touristy places, so we could at least get out and do something worth crossing the ocean for! It wasn't going to be what I had planned, but I decided I would be happy to at least have them near enough to hug goodnight and not talk to them through a phone or Skype.

My father, on the other hand, had been truly changed by this journey of faith we were embarking on with Caleb. He boldly said he was praying that they would get to come home with us. I had my doubts. Not doubts of Caleb's healing, but of leaving the hospital anytime soon. The doctors had made it clear that with just the damage already done, we weren't going anywhere for a long time. One doctor had even jokingly commented that we would "become like the furniture in the hospital." My dad permitted me to book new lodging and change their plane reservations, but he still believed the vacation he had planned for so long would go on in Gaborone as he had pictured it. He knew that the God who was so good to promise Caleb's healing wasn't going to let him cross an ocean and not hold his precious little grandchildren in his arms.

However, within the week, our hopes, unexpectedly, began to rise. By the end of the second week, Caleb was doing so well that to my surprise the neurologist began talking of a possibility of being released that coming Sunday. My parents were due to arrive that coming Saturday. I was afraid to get excited because I didn't want to be too disappointed. The early release depended entirely on the second brain scans. Had God truly healed Caleb's brain? Would we see different scans and be released that soon? I could only dream that He would be so merciful!

Chapter Nine

Drowning in doubts

Friday, the long awaited test day, arrived. Caleb was scheduled to have an eye test, a hearing test, and his second M.R.I. The E.E.G. test results would be ready as well. The hope of an early discharge depended on these outcomes. Yes, Friday was a big day! Percy and I were like giddy school children waiting to get back a test we knew we had aced! We had experienced God in the quiet of our hearts. By the end of that day, we hoped we wouldn't be the only ones experiencing God! With those scans and test results, we hoped to have physical evidence of God's miraculous healing in Caleb's brain.

The minutes trickled by painfully slowly. How much longer until someone would walk in holding Caleb's test results? We hovered by the door, hearts leaping every time it swung open. The nurses laughed at our comical jitters.

Finally, the door opened, and a doctor holding a file marked with Caleb's name passed by. It was the ophthalmologist. We rushed over to hear his findings. "I'm sorry," were his first words. What!? Those weren't the words we wanted to hear. We wearily took our seats as the doctor continued... due to the extreme trauma of his birth, his eyes were still full of blood. They couldn't even see the back of his eye to determine whether he had vision. All they could see was blood and deducted that is all our precious boy could see as well. The medical term used to describe his condition was sub retinal hemorrhaging with swelling at the optical nerve. Imagine, all along we thought little Caleb had been looking in our eyes and watching our smiles. It was just an illusion. What our boy had seen for the past two weeks was nothing but blood. The ophthalmologist reassured us that in time the blood would be absorbed, but the more important unanswerable question still loomed ahead. Would he be blind? Only time would tell. For now, one thing was certain. Caleb had failed his eye test.

The first good news came next. Caleb passed his hearing test! At least he could hear. That was something to smile about, but I still couldn't push the possibility of Caleb being blind out of my mind. Just then the neurologist walked through the door holding Caleb's brain scans. He motioned for us to the white board with the light at the back so we could clearly see the scans. Surely, this, too, was going to be good news. We hurried over.

The neurologist inspected us, as if sizing us up on our ability to handle the news. Then those dreaded words came again, "I am sorry, but nothing has changed." He quickly added that the good news, in his opinion, was that the brain was healing so there wasn't any further damage being done. Nonetheless, the brain damage caused by his birth was permanent.

Permanent? No! Still clinging to the hope of a miracle, I said, "If it is healing, isn't that a good thing?"

He explained, "Most tissues in the body regenerate when they heal. For example, if I get a cut on my hand, the tissue will actually heal, and in time, I wouldn't be able to detect where I had been cut. Unfortunately, the brain is an internal organ which never regenerates."

He went on to tell us that the right frontal lobe was gone. It didn't even show up on a scan. In its place was a black hole. Most likely, it wouldn't be functional at all. The left occipital lobe was also mostly gone. And there were several patches that had been severely deprived of oxygen. The dominant one was located in the left hemisphere. The scan showed an obvious streak that ran upwards through that left side. He showed us several other areas that had been damaged but said that the concentration of the damage was in those three areas.

"So, what does this mean?" I questioned. He patiently smiled and said he wasn't a prophet and couldn't predict the future. Well, that didn't answer my question! I wanted facts. I wanted to know exactly what we were dealing with here! I pushed and finally he conceded, explaining that the brain is a mysterious organ. Two people with exactly the same injury could be affected in totally different ways. He gave us an example. One child, lacking this frontal lobe, could be extremely docile, another extremely agitated and impossible to calm. We should be grateful, he encouraged, because it seemed Caleb was showing signs towards the calmer child.

The fact was that the frontal lobe determined Caleb's personality. It would enable him, the doctor clarified, to have memories, to discern right from wrong, to have impulse control, and to concentrate. He expounded on this with another example. A man without that frontal lobe may see a pretty lady and just shout out his raw thoughts at her. Basically, without the frontal lobe, Caleb could mature outwardly, but we would still have to treat him like a child. He wouldn't know whether he could cross a road safely or how to interact in normal social environments.

That was not all. The left occipital lobe, which was also severely damaged, determines vision, mainly peripheral vision. Even if Caleb's eyes healed up from the blood damage, his brain may not have the ability to communicate with his eyes to allow them to see. Or, the double whammy was that his vision could be affected in both his brain and in his literal eye with the optical nerve damage. The large damaged streak that ran across his left hemisphere would most likely affect his ability to have purposeful movements with his right side as well. He didn't think he would be paralyzed, but he would lack the ability to have planned purposeful movements, like holding a pen or eating with a utensil.

At worst-case scenario, we were looking at a blind child who could neither write his name nor eat his own food and would be under our care indefinitely because he couldn't discern right from wrong in order to operate normally in the world.

The report from the E.E.G. test was a bit better. He said low delta waves in the back of the brain showed that it was still sick but it didn't show sharp spikes which would indicate seizures. In layman's terms, it wasn't healed yet, but it was getting there. It looked like the seizures were stopping.

I sat stupefied, not even able to cry. I was so sure that this scan was going to be different. I was so sure I had heard God say He was going to heal Caleb.

We thanked the doctor and mechanically wandered over to Caleb's bed.

He laid there the same as always except... wait. His feeding tube was back in his nose. We called the nurse over. "Why does he have the feeding tube? I thought he was exclusively on the bottle now." She sorrowfully recounted that he had vomited after every feeding that day. It was essential that he eat and the tube was the only way to ensure he kept his food down. It didn't look like we were going home on Sunday after all.

Discouragement dampened our every step as we journeyed to our room. I collapsed against Percy's chest. What was I thinking believing God could heal him? We had been told repeatedly that brain damage is permanent. I felt like Peter. He had walked on water, believing the impossible, as he fixed his eyes on Jesus. When the storm roared angrily around him, though, he sunk. That was me. It was too much. I felt like the waves were crashing in on me; I too was sinking. I couldn't believe in the impossible. Facts were facts. People don't walk on water and brains don't heal themselves.

Percy, on the other hand, was surer than ever of what he had heard. He held me tightly as I sobbed and then cupped my face up so he could look me in the eyes. "Ashley," he whispered steadfastly, "Hope in the Lord does not disappoint. His promises are yes and amen in Christ. Cling to His promise. Walk in faith and not by sight." It was too late for that. I was drowning in my doubts.

Chapter Ten

He gives life to the dead

"Percy", I muttered, "please, may I be alone?" Alone, amongst the shadows of my room, something broke inside me. I laid weeping, and weeping, and weeping some more. I felt so stupid that I had been so naïve as to believe that God could heal Caleb. My poor baby silently suffered and there wasn't anything I could do. Even our prayers hadn't changed his situation. Hopelessness was closing in around me like the dark shadows on the walls. I had to pull myself together. How? Tears crusted on my cheeks. I heaved myself off the bed and into my wheelchair. "Could someone assist me to the maternity ward," I inquired at the front desk using the room's phone. Maybe a hot bath was what I needed.

Meanwhile, after leaving me, Percy slipped into the N.I.C.U., seated himself closely next to his beloved son and stalwartly began reading God's word into Caleb's hearing ears and his own aching heart. My husband was the standard bearer for our family.

I, on the other hand, sunk down deep into the soothing hot salted bath. I splashed my tear stained cheeks and breathed deeply; deep enough, hopefully, to release all the hovering anxieties and fears that still lurked all around me. No, the day had not gone like I expected. It had been too much for me to bear. I reached over the side of the tub for my Bible. "God, would you please comfort me through your word? I need it so much."

I flipped through and read random passages. Nothing changed. I still felt despondent. Then, my eyes fell on a passage I didn't think I had seen before.

If I had read it, I hadn't thought much about it, at least not until today. I read Romans 4:17-21. It described Abraham, and how he believed that God could give them a child, even though Sarah's womb was as good as dead. He claimed that God gave life to the dead and called things that were not as though they were. The passage said Abraham faced the facts yet did not waver regarding the promise he had received. He was fully persuaded that God had the power to do what He had promised.

I scooted up in the tub and opened the door a crack with my fingers, scanning the room. Good, there was no one in the room. I didn't want someone to think I was crazy if they heard me talking to myself in the bathtub. I decided to substitute my name in the verse and read it aloud. Here is what I said. "He is the God who gives life to the dead and calls things that are not as though they are. Against all hope, Ashley and Percy, in hope, believed. Without weakening in our faith, we faced the fact that Caleb's brain is as good as dead in some areas. Yet, we do not waver through unbelief regarding the promise of God, but are strengthened in our faith and give glory to God, being fully persuaded that God has the power to do what He has promised!!"

I must have repeated that verse twenty times until every moral fiber in my body owned it, fully possessed it. No more doubts or hesitations. No more qualms or misgivings. That verse lived in me. It was my personal truth. I CAN face the facts BUT I will NOT waver in my faith. God CAN give life to the dead and I AM persuaded that He has the power to do what He promised! Relief flooded my inner soul. God hadn't abandoned me. He could still work a miracle in Caleb. He WOULD still work a miracle in Caleb. Joy bubbled up in me again. No, the day hadn't turned out the way I had envisioned, but the Lord was true to His promise in 1 Corinthians 10:13. He had NOT given me too much to bear. I thought Caleb's second scans were going to be different. But, just because the scans weren't different didn't mean God wasn't at work. It just meant He was doing it in His timing and in His way instead of mine!

I heard a soft knock on the door. "Ashley?" Percy whispered. "Are you in there? I know you said you wanted to be alone, but I need to share something that God just showed me." I told him to enter. He opened his Bible and my mouth dropped.

He began to read Romans 4:17-21! He even substituted our names like I had done. I kept quiet as he read. Then, when he finished and geared up to encourage me out of my "pit of despair," I began to chuckle! "Oh, God is soo good Percy." I told him of what God had just taught me. Some might call it a coincidence but we knew differently. Out of the thousands of verses we both could have read, we knew it had to be God that we learned the same lesson, with the same passage of scripture, in two different places at the same time. It was no coincidence in our minds! Before that day, I honestly don't recall ever reading Romans 4:17-21. After that day, I knew I would never forget it!

We weren't sure what God had up His sleeve. Unquestionably, though, we knew that Caleb's healing was still a go! He had given us our Rhema, His spoken word for us, to cling to and claim in the weeks and months to come.

Scripture declares in Psalms 30:5 that tears may come at night but joy comes in the morning. We experienced this truth as we woke up with joy on Saturday morning. I was like a little girl on Christmas Eve counting down the hours until Christmas morning. Today was the day I would see my parents. I still wasn't sure if we would be spending their vacation time here at the hospital or back home, but at that point I didn't care. The hours couldn't pass fast enough. I couldn't wait to see them!

There was rejoicing in Caleb's room as well. His feeding tube was gone. One of the nurses had suggested adding a thickening agent in his bottle to help keep his milk down. It worked, and he was back on the bottle. I was so optimistic that I even requested another go at breastfeeding him at the next feeding. They hesitantly agreed.

The next feeding arrived. Since there is no way to measure how much milk a child takes while breastfeeding, the nurses weighed him. They would weigh him before and after breastfeeding. Assuming everything but the amount of milk remained the same, it should give an accurate idea of the amount of milk he ingested. The nurse helped find a suitable position to facilitate feeding Caleb. They had him on a schedule to eat every three hours. To minimize fatigue, he had thirty minutes to finish the feeding. If I couldn't successfully feed him in 20 minutes, they would use the remaining ten minutes to give him a bottle. As his lips began to smack, they set the timer. The timer rang signaling 20 minutes had elapsed. They put him on the scale. Nothing had changed! No way, I thought! Their scales must be wrong! She insisted the scales were fine, and I needed to give up my hopes of breastfeeding Caleb. I stood firm. Article after article I'd read showed that research had proven there are numerous benefits to breastfeeding. Caleb needed all the help he could get. This was the only area I had any control over helping him, and I desired so much to give him this gift.

The nurse kindly responded that she understood my heart but unless she was convinced that Caleb would receive adequate nutrition, she couldn't in good conscience release him. If I were to agree to bottle feeding, all signs pointed to his release tomorrow, Sunday. The pediatrician came by on his morning rounds and also agreed that unless things changed, he didn't see any reason Caleb couldn't be released the next day. I literally jumped up and down!! I still had this grand maternal instinct to breastfeed, but my desire to take my baby home was greater. Seeing my obvious excitement, she was quick to bring me back to earth. "Now, remember," she cautioned. "We are releasing him because he no longer needs the aid of the machines here to live. It does not mean he is healed. He is still a very sick boy with major brain damage."

I didn't even care. God was going to heal him! I was going home, and my parents should be there any minute! I was on cloud nine!

Optimism ran thick. When my parents got there, we asked a huge favor. "Is it possible for my parents to hold Caleb?" Wow, they lifted Caleb from his web of wires, took him into a little waiting area within the N.I.C.U. and my parents held their grandson for the first time. They just stared at him in wonder. For three weeks they had heard all about baby Caleb, now he lay peacefully in their arms.

"He's perfect," my mom gushed.

"He looks totally normal," my dad observed. I could tell they were wondering what the fuss was about. Caleb did look fine. I had to remind them that brain damage was different than other illnesses. It would not be evident for years to come. When all the other babies started to walk, a child with Caleb's brain damage may limp if he could even walk. When all the other kids began memorizing their alphabet and concentrating on what the teacher was teaching them, a child with Caleb's brain wouldn't be able to participate. When it came time to drive a car, a child with Caleb's brain wouldn't be allowed behind a wheel. He would lack the proper eye sight to see the road clearly. With or without a miracle, Caleb looked normal now because he was a newborn. The evidence of God's healing hand on Caleb's life would be visible if he met normal childhood developmental milestones.

Chapter Eleven

Bittersweet freedom

Sunday morning was bittersweet.

Unitas hospital had been our refuge for almost three weeks. Within the comfort of its shielding walls, we were immunized from both the regular routines or life and its harsh realities. Our sole responsibilities consisted of loving Caleb and seeking God. Percy didn't work. A maid cleaned our room. At meal times, prepared food was brought and placed on our laps and when we finished, it magically disappeared. In addition, if Caleb had a seizure, they put on the oxygen mask and intervened immediately. If Caleb couldn't keep his food down, they put a tube down his throat, sending nutrients directly to his stomach. If his oxygen levels changed, an alarm went off. If the emotional drain left us exhausted, we hung our "do not disturb" sign on the door and slept. We slept until refreshment woke us up, knowing the nurses, ever ready, bathed, fed, and vigilantly attended our son. Yes, the hospital was our refuge and we were grateful refugees.

On this day, however, all that was going to change. We were commencing to walk out of our sanctuary and enter reality. Our world had abruptly changed. What would it look like for us outside these walls? I was going to be responsible for our little guy. Caleb still had never cried or uttered a sound so if something went wrong, I had no way of knowing. He needed a round-the-clock sentinel discerning his problems. Come Monday, Percy returned to work and I was going home to a 22-month-old baby girl who hadn't had my attention in three weeks. Realistically, I couldn't be at Caleb's side at all hours of the day. I had other responsibilities that couldn't be put on hold forever to give him constant care. It was intimidating. Yes, I longed to be home, but home wasn't the same anymore. Could I really do this?

The nurses laughed at my apprehension. "Remember, this is what you were jumping up and down about the other day," they kindly chided.

Nevertheless, they understood my hesitation. They turned my last morning into a crash course for living with a brain injured child. Percy and I had to watch videos teaching us how to do infant CPR, to watch for signs of dehydration, and to know how to take his temperature. We were educated on different symptoms to look for and given a list of which ones were life threatening and which ones we could treat at home. They advised us to buy an apnea mat that would sound an alarm if Caleb stopped breathing; then they trained us how to use it. They showed us what to do if he started convulsing. I had to practice putting the thickening agent in his milk and gave him a bottle under their supervision. Our heads spun from the overload, but there was still more information to cram.

They reminded us that although they rejoiced with us that Caleb was well enough to be released, his journey to recovery was far from over. They gave us a list of milestones that a normal baby should hit by certain ages. At any stage, should we realize he wasn't progressing properly, we should take him to a doctor. From there, we would decide on the best course of action depending on the physician's advice. Some things could be improved with early intervention of occupational and physical therapy, and some things, they counseled, would never develop and would forever remind us of the brain loss he had suffered.

Finally, I scheduled a 4-month follow up appointment with the pediatric neurologist. I was urged to locate a competent Gaborone pediatrician along with an ophthalmologist and occupational therapist – all right away!

We signed his discharge papers and the anticipated moment arrived. It was time to go. The nurses unhooked Caleb from all the machines and we carried him out. A friend from Percy's work had driven down from Botswana to pick all of us up. He waited patiently in the car park. We strapped Caleb in a car seat. Then, we began the seemingly impossible task of fitting all my parent's luggage plus all the things we had accumulated in the car. Afterwards, my parents, Percy, and I tried to find space, which was a challenge since the luggage seemed to ooze out of every nook and cranny of the car. Finally, we all squished in and got situated for the long drive ahead of us.

I had a portable pump and expressed the milk in the car to give Caleb. When the liquid reached the designated mark on the bottle, we pulled over at a shopping mall and fed him. We also grabbed some fast food and were off again. Only an hour later did I realize that I had forgotten to put the thickening agent in his milk. Surprisingly, he had not thrown up. In the hospital, he threw up without the thickener. By accident, he took a bottle without the thickener and kept it down. It was a little thing but it showed God was healing him bit by bit.

For the most part, the drive home was uneventful as Caleb slept most of the way. Eventually, roads started to look familiar and I knew we were getting close. As we crossed the border, I couldn't wait any longer. I had to hear my little princess's voice. We called Dana, our friend who was keeping Anna Catherine, to let her know we were near hoping that if she left her house right then, we would arrive at our home around the same time. I didn't want to be at my house and not have my little girl in my arms!

We turned the corner and drove up my street. Were all those cars at my house? I had given the house keys to my friend, Simone, when we left. She had let herself in and transformed my dining room into an elegant dinner setting. A home cooked meal steamed on the table; fresh flowers brightened the room; my good china dishes shone against the lacey white table cloth while praise music softly played in the background. My friend had all the lights on and had even rearranged some furniture, making my house look magnificent! My mom was more than impressed; I beamed with pride. She approved! Again, it was a small thing; but God had provided yet another small desire of mine. Everything combined for an unforgettable welcome home. Even our friends gathered at the door to greet us. But as I took this glorious site in, I still felt pangs of disappointment. My spunky little girl was nowhere to be seen.

Caleb was asleep when we arrived. We carried him into our bedroom and left him sleeping in his car seat so not to disturb him from the party in the other room.

As we settled, a car drove up. My cute little girl bounced out of the door, ran up the driveway, and sprung into my arms. Finally, things were complete. After a long hug, she stood back and started spilling story after story of all her adventures. My world was looking up. My parents were there. My daughter was cuddling up in my arms. My friends had shown overwhelming support and thoughtfulness. I had a hot meal on my table that I didn't have to cook. I smiled. God was good!

Suddenly, a few of us heard a funny noise. What was that? I listened again and thought it must be those neighborhood cats fighting because it sounded like a shrill cry. It happened again, and we all got quiet. It was coming from my bedroom. I rushed back to find Caleb screaming in his car seat. Normally, a mother would feel guilty to know her baby was in the room crying while she was out mingling with her friends, but not me! I was elated. Caleb was three weeks old and he had just uttered his first cry! God was good!

Anna Cathrine loves her new baby brother

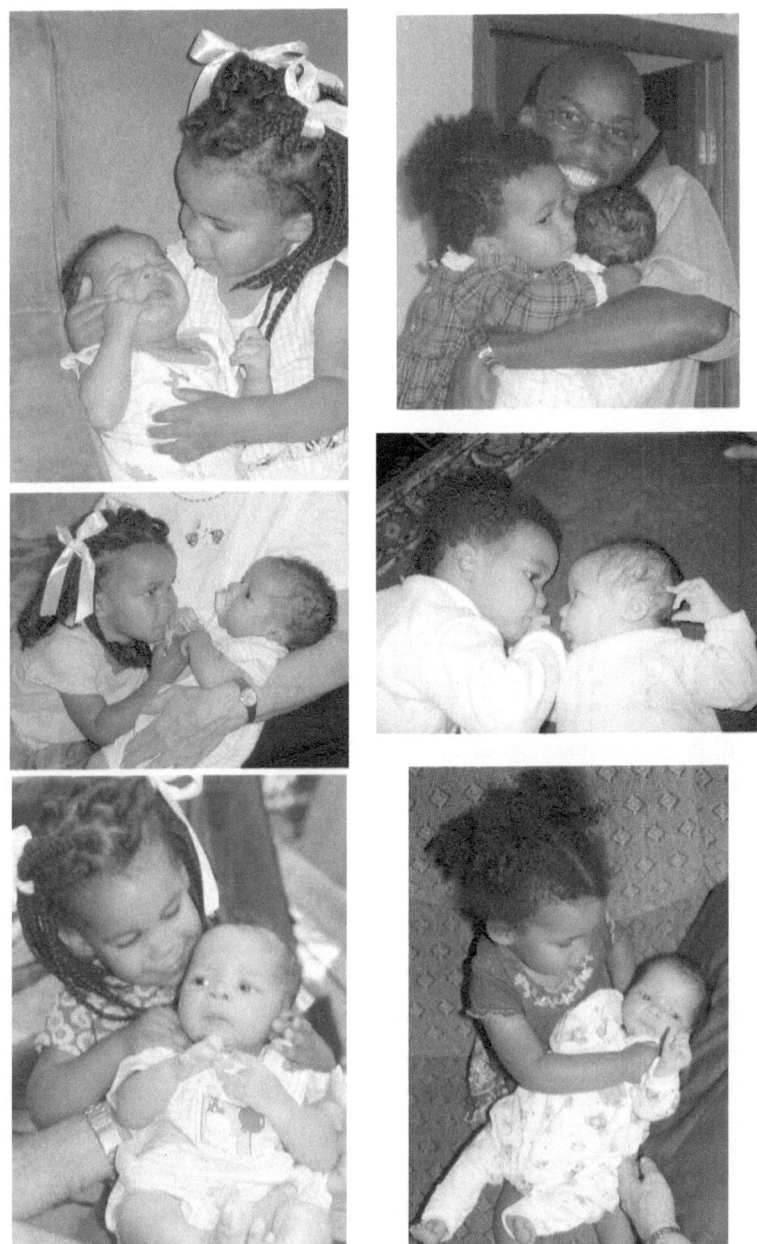

Chapter Twelve

Coming home

Strangely, my "can-I-do-this" apprehensions vanished when we got home. The first night I had anticipated, literally, standing over the bed watching him in fear that something would go wrong. On the contrary, I didn't even bother to unpack the apnea mat we had spent so much money buying. Something inside me just knew he would be okay. We laid him in his crib and went to bed. I now knew he could cry if he was hungry. I didn't set an alarm. I knew his internal clock would tell me. For me, I would just sleep like any mother of a newborn, with my ears perked ready to spring out of bed at any moment.

The first week home I dutifully followed all the precautionary orders. I gave Caleb my expressed breast milk in a bottle without trying to breastfeed him directly. I looked for a pediatrician. I took him to an ophthalmologist. I couldn't find an occupational therapist in our city but I found a physical therapist and made the appointment. One thing I didn't do, however, was bother opening the apnea mat. I am not sure why, because it couldn't have hurt. But, for some reason, every time I went to open it, I felt God assuring me I didn't need it. He didn't slumber, and He would watch over our son even when I couldn't.

I checked out several pediatricians, but none of them seemed like the right fit. I wanted someone who was interested in Caleb's history and was knowledgeable in brain damage. I had lots of questions and knew as time went on, I would have many more. I wanted someone who would take the time to listen to my concerns and answer my questions in such a way that I could understand medically what was going on with my son. After a few different visits, I gave up and rationalized that if Caleb was sick, at least I knew where I could find them.

I went to the ophthalmologist. Blood still filled Caleb's eyes. She verified that the blood would most likely dissolve, but she wasn't sure what the lasting damage would be. She encouraged me to come back in a couple of weeks; but, it had been such a headache to make this first appointment, drive across town, and sit in her waiting room for almost two hours. I just figured since she had said presently, there was nothing she could do, I would let nature run its course and save our money and time on continued visits.

The physical therapist was next on the calendar. She was the nicest of all the different medical people I visited that week. I liked her immediately! She had an obvious interest in Caleb and a love for her work; but as I watched her do different movements with Caleb, I thought, I could do those at home. How much therapy could one really do with a newborn? I would intentionally play with him and stimulate him like any good mother then go back when he was older. Maybe then she could offer specific exercises that wouldn't come naturally to me without having any professional training in children's therapy.

Other than visiting multiple doctors, my parents' visit went pretty much as I had dreamed. We went on a game drive viewing the famous African wildlife. My dad treated us to dinners at delicious fancy restaurants. They enjoyed the all-you-can-eat meat dinner at a local Brazilian restaurant and the succulent fresh fish dish served at an upper class golf estate restaurant. Since Caleb was bottle-fed, my mom was able to help with a lot of the night time feedings. My parents doted on their beloved grandchildren, even buying Anna Catherine and Caleb a swing set as an early Christmas present since they didn't know when they would see the kids again. Percy's parents took advantage of the rare chance to meet my parents and travelled the 6 hour drive from their home in northern Botswana to meet my mom and dad and hold their first grandson in their arms. The only thing I hadn't planned on was that our church family dropped by so often to see us and pray over Caleb that it didn't leave much quality time to spend with my parents. We stayed busy entertaining all our concerned friends. However, my mom and dad were blessed to see how loved we were and how prayed over Caleb was. But as the saying goes, all good things must come to an end. After three weeks, we had to say good bye, sadly, not knowing when we would see them again.

At first, I pictured my calendar filled with Caleb's doctor appointments.

However, as time wore on, I just didn't see the need. All I did was spend a lot of money and time in waiting rooms to be told what I already knew. Repeatedly, I was reminded that with brain damage or even the eye damage, at Caleb's young age, there was really nothing they could do. So I stopped going. Sometimes I felt guilty for not taking him to see doctors more regularly, but then I would just remind myself that they couldn't change Caleb. Only God had the power to do that.

By the second week, I got more daring. Against, the hospital's advice, I tried breastfeeding again. Pumping milk and giving it to him in a bottle was getting old fast! I knew all the reasons I wasn't supposed to breastfeed. He would never have the strength to suckle so I shouldn't tire him out. Still, it couldn't hurt to try just once more. I started off with only one of his 7-8 daily feedings. I rationalized if he didn't eat enough at that feeding, he would just take in more at the next. After all, he was eating every three hours. He wasn't going to starve. I didn't have the fancy scale they used before and after breast feedings in N.I.C.U.. Instead, I used motherly logic learned from my experiences. If he cried, he was hungry; if he didn't, he was full. After the first attempt and my well calculated observations, I deduced success and added another breastfeeding. Within 3 weeks after being discharged, Caleb was doing what the nurses had said would most likely be impossible. He was exclusively breastfeeding.

I finally made the trip I was dreading. I went down to our medical aid to reconcile the bills. We needed to know our outstanding balance. As I suspected, the bills were astronomical, but, surprisingly, I wasn't worried. Somehow, God filled me with the assurance He would provide. Sure enough, around the globe God began laying our financial burden on people's hearts. College sorority sisters donated. The church plant I was a part of in Canada gave. People from my prayer team called my father and inquired how they could deposit money into our account. Before we knew it, astronomical bills dwindled to zero. In the end, our personal, out-of-pocket expenses turned out to be around what we had saved in planning for the normal private hospital delivery. At every turn, God was demonstrating to us that He was trustworthy.

As time passed, a vital part of my self-imposed job included studying Caleb. I noticed he favored lying on his left side. He even struggled to look at a movement on his right side. Therefore, every time I laid him down, I intentionally put him on his right side. I put toys in his bed on the right side. I made fast movements on his right side to try and entice him to turn his head. Slowly, we saw a change. After a couple of months, a stranger wouldn't have been able to tell which side he favored. As he started to play with toys, again I noticed that he never used his right hand. I held his left hand and forced him to use the right hand. It was hard work because he fought me and cried. It was obvious he didn't want to use that right side, but I enforced these little exercises daily. He also took his left hand and played with his left foot, but he never played with his right foot. Consequently, I added baby calisthenics to our daily routine, stretching each hand separately diagonally across his midline to touch the opposite foot.

Other than the obvious preferred use of his left side, Caleb seemed like any other normal baby. He even excelled in some areas! By nine weeks, he was sleeping all night! He was gaining weight and by five weeks, he even began to smile at me. At first, I refused to let myself get excited, rationalizing it was that gas smile that mothers talk about. But as it became more common, I knew he was actually smiling. Did that mean he could see me?

By November, he was cooing and saying "ga ga" like all other two-month-old babies. In general, he was content and happy. He rarely cried and was a pure delight to have around. Something else remarkable began happening in November. He began batting toys under his hanging mobile. I knew he could see, but I decided it wouldn't hurt to confirm it with an ophthalmologist. She examined his eyes, did a few tests and confirmed my suspicions. Caleb could see. She still warned that with the damage to the occipital lobe, we should expect that he would have problems seeing anything in his peripheral vision, but at his age, it would be impossible to test that. It would be another two years at least before we could truly know whether he could see in that manner. For now, we rejoiced that he had functional frontal vision.

As the November calendar flipped over to December, Caleb flipped right along with it. He began flipping regularly from his stomach to his back. When lying flat on his stomach, he could look up and hold his head steady for a substantial amount of time. One day, in church, I looked over at a friend of mine who was holding Caleb. Caleb was flashing her one of his adorable gummy grins, but tears were streaming down her face. I whispered, "What's wrong?"

She gushed, " I was looking at him now, remembering what he looked like when the medical rescue men wheeled him off at the hospital in that incubator after he was born. God is soo good! This is more than we could have ever dreamed, having seen how bad he was at birth!"

As the months went by, I posted pictures of Caleb on our family website. Emails kept popping up in my inbox with testimonies of how people's faith had been strengthened by following Caleb's story and seeing his pictures. It was humbling to know God was using our little man to lead people around the world to give Him glory and draw them closer to Him. All I could do was join them in praising God!

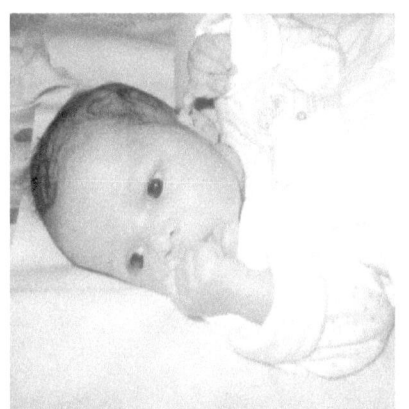

Caleb, on his first night at home from hospital

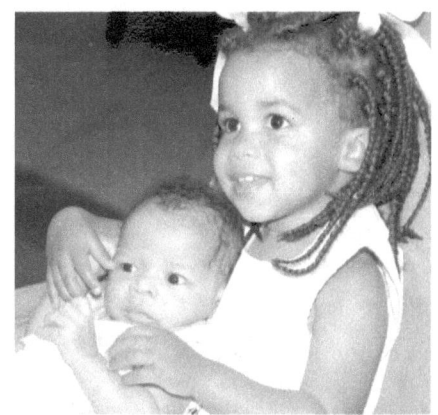

Anna Catherine and Caleb, 5 weeks old

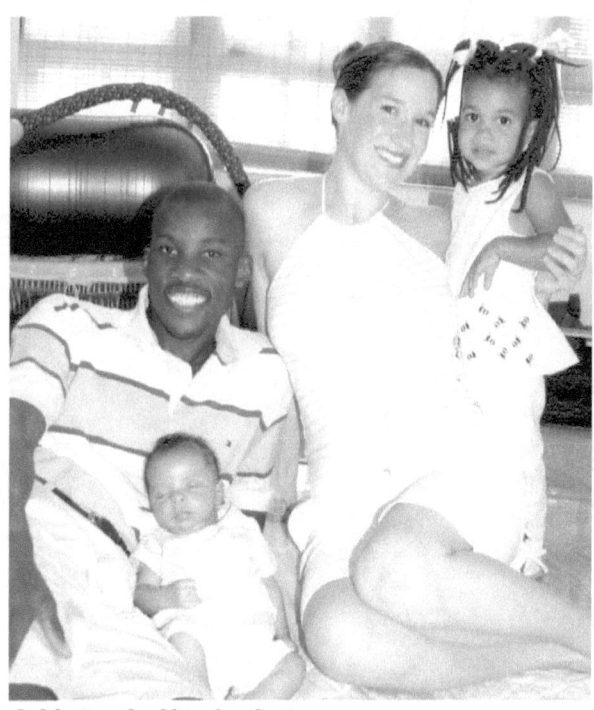

Caleb, 5 weeks old, in family picture

Anna Catherine and Celeb's Grandparents

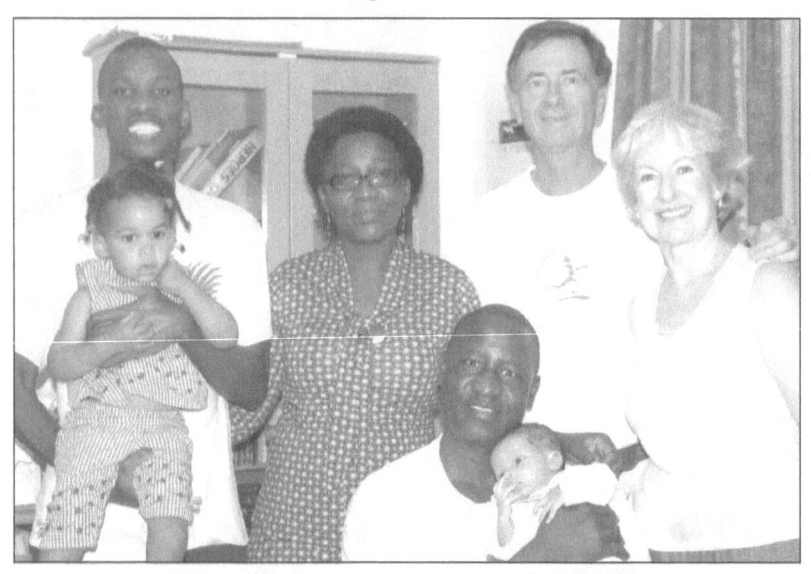

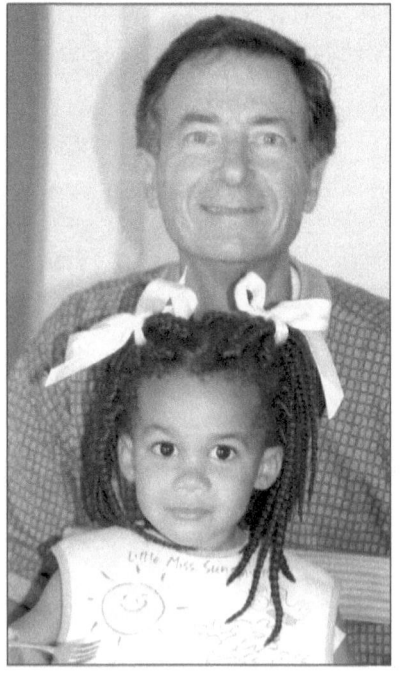

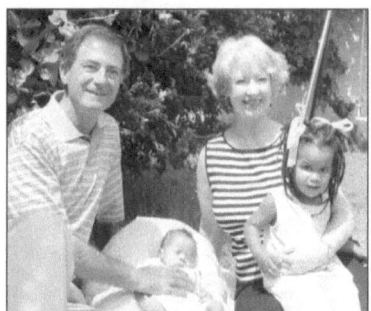

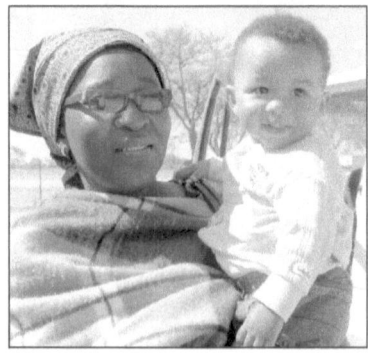

Chapter Thirteen

… and it will be yours

January was around the corner. We were scheduled to go back to Pretoria to meet with the pediatric neurologist for Caleb's four month check up. By our observations, he was doing so well that we weren't keen on spending more money and time on the long trip. Nevertheless, we felt it was the responsible thing to do. We arranged for a babysitter for Anna Catherine again and headed back to South Africa. Caleb was becoming quite the international traveler!

Before Caleb's check up, the doctor requested a referral for another M.R.I., Caleb's third one in his short existence. The referral read like the memory of a bad dream: "severe birth asphyxia survivor with Right frontal traumatic hematoma and subdural hemorrhages. Need drainage??" Survivor? That word sounded so serious. It was hard to believe that was Caleb's history four months ago when he was doing so well now.

As we waited for the results, we walked around our old "home." There were many familiar faces. The more shocking fact was how many of them still remembered us. Thousands of people must walk in and out and of that hospital daily, yet person after person kept coming up and asking about Caleb by name! We were humbled! One lady even asked if she could take a picture of him with her cell phone. She said she and her coworker had often talked about us and wondered what had happened with Caleb. She said she needed to show her a picture because her coworker wasn't going to believe it was the same child! Another lady literally ran up and hugged us. Her whole church had been praying for us, and she couldn't wait to tell them of his outstanding progress. Even the guard posted at the door timidly remarked he remembered us. Once again, we had an opportunity to share the incredible story of our little breathing miracle. God received much glory that day as He shone brightly out of our infant son.

²⁴Therefore I tell you, whatever you ask for in prayer, believe that you have received it, and it will be yours." (Mark 11:24 NIV) Just four months earlier, we had boldly asked God for healing in this same place. God had kept His end of the deal and had given us more than we could have imagined in our journey of faith!

Finally, the M.R.I. results were ready. Results in hand, Percy, Caleb and I met with the pediatric neurologist. He studied the scans and again repeated that nothing had changed. In fact, the empty cavity in the right frontal lobe had actually filled with water. The entire left hemisphere had shrunk due to the damage, and the left occipital was still severely compromised. His tragic birth had indeed caused permanent damage to his brain.

However, after physically examining Caleb, he smiled and shook his head. If he hadn't personally seen this child in a life threatening state four months earlier, he declared, he would doubt these scans went with this child. He did all kinds of tests and finally proclaimed that his milestone development was miraculous! Of course, we had already been rejoicing in our little miracle boy, but what an encouragement to hear a doctor who daily studied brain damage and the effects on children to authenticate it! After concluding the examination, the doctor said there wasn't one milestone he expected Caleb to be at by that age that hadn't been reached. "He is perfect!" said the neurologist with confidence. Then, jokingly he added that if we didn't want Caleb, he would take him because he seemed like such a happy, healthy baby. After giving us time to celebrate, he added that the brain damage was extensive and was worried that Caleb may start having seizures again. He also warned that although he couldn't prophesy the future, injuries like Caleb's typically resulted in concentration and memory difficulties in school. He concluded our meeting with one last piece of information. Caleb, most like, wouldn't have peripheral vision and possibly may not be able to make purposeful movements with his right side.

It was a very expensive, time consuming visit to tell us what we already knew, but we were happy we went. Now it was clear it wasn't just a biased parent's perspective. A doctor had confirmed that Caleb's improvement was, in his words, miraculous! Yes, we knew he wasn't perfect yet, per se, but we clung to the same faith that led Paul to write Philippians 1:6. We were confident that He who had begun a good work in Caleb would carry it on to completion. If God could partially heal, why not go all the way? If He could create Caleb, then surely fixing that which He created was far easier than forming him from nothing in my womb. We rejoiced in the good news of the day and in faith believed that it was just the beginning of a long line of positive doctors' reports.

We danced in the car all the way back to Botswana, singing praise songs and thanking God for His healing touch on our son!

Shortly after Caleb was born, we had been asked to give a testimony in our church. Our local church in Botswana had walked closely in prayer with us throughout our entire time in South Africa yet most of them had never seen Caleb. They wanted to see the object of their prayers and hear an update directly from us. We had declared in front of hundreds of people that we were resting in the promise that God would heal Caleb. At that time, we had no physical evidence of any kind of healing. He was just a newborn and all newborns, brain damaged or not, mainly just lie there. Now that he was older and we had a doctor's report stating his phenomenal improvement, we were asked to speak again.

I wrote the following in a prayer letter asking my prayer team to pray for Percy as he spoke.

*Percy has been asked to give a follow-up testimony this Sunday at our church, Open Baptist. The verses that come to our mind are John 10:10 and Revelation 12:10. John tells us that the thief comes to steal, kill, and destroy but God has come so that we may have abundant life. Although Satan may have had plans to hurt or even kill Caleb, we believe that God has plans to give him life and life to the full! Scripture says in Revelation 12:10 that the devil accuses us and hurls insults at us. In this instance, they look something like this: "His brain is severely damaged... you are crazy to believe God can heal that. You are insane to not be angry and sue those doctors. You better not say it out loud that you believe God can heal, because if he doesn't, you are going to look like a fool." That same scripture in Revelation goes on to say "They **overcame him** by the blood of the Lamb and by the word of their testimony."* We will continue to joyfully say out loud that our faith is in the GREAT PHYSICIAN, our Lord and our Savior! We can overcome these negative thoughts that Satan accuses us with by the blood of the Lamb and the words that come out of our mouth! Pray that God uses Percy this week to encourage others to claim God's words and to PROCLAIM God's promises over the trials of their lives!

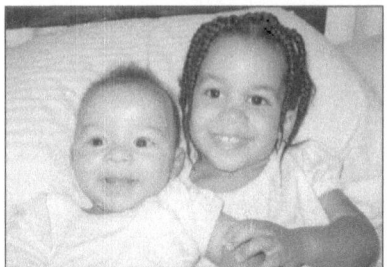

A.C. and Caleb, 3 months

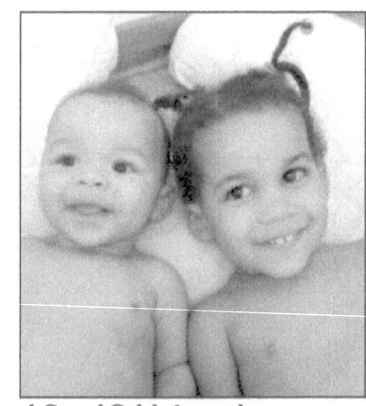

A.C. and Caleb, 3 months

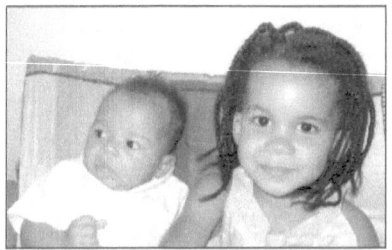

A.C. and Caleb, 2 months

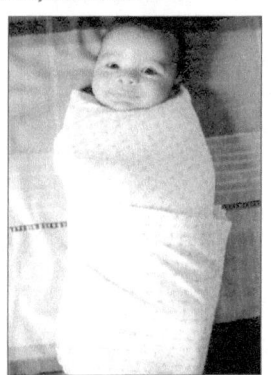

Caleb, 1 month

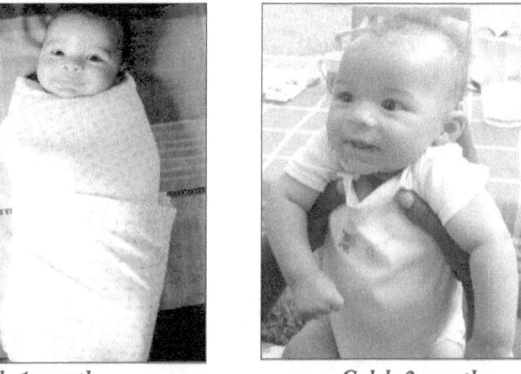

Caleb, 2 months

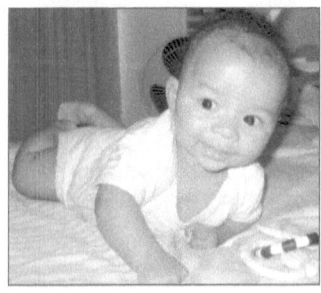

Caleb, 3 months

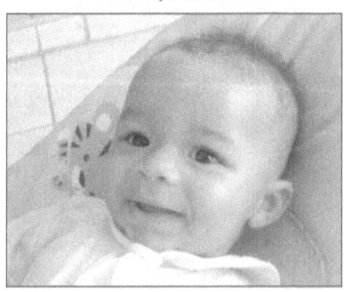

Caleb, 4 months

Chapter Fourteen

Help my unbelief

Percy's testimony went great. People's tears, smiles, and hugs made it obvious they sympathetically walked this journey with us. We were eternally grateful for the love and support our church family continued to offer.

Time passed, and Caleb continued to improve. My calendar diary recorded on January 27, 2010, at 4 months and 3 weeks old, Caleb sat independently for a whole 5 minutes! He hit that milestone ahead of Anna Catherine and she had been advanced in all her motor skills. In my eyes, that was major. In order to sit balanced, both sides of the body had to be communicating with the brain. It wasn't a fine motor skill like buttoning a button, but it was still another reason to rejoice! He was progressing nicely!

In February, I had a unique opportunity to accompany Percy on a business trip to Cape Town, South Africa. Because Caleb was still exclusively breastfed, he had to go with us. Percy's work mates called him the "conference mascot." People marveled over how calm and smiley he was and how he never cried. Men took pictures with Caleb to show their wives back home that there was a baby that didn't cry when they picked him up. Ladies asked in advance if they could hold him during lunch or breaks. He truly was unbelievable. We didn't mention his tragic past. No one would have guessed it anyway. He looked and seemed like the perfect baby!

By March, he was flipping from his back to his stomach, another milestone he hit before his sister! However, something was starting to bother me. My calendar revealed by six months Anna Catherine had been crawling and even balancing on her knees to play with toys in both hands. Caleb was six months and wasn't crawling, neither forwards and backwards. When I voiced my concerns to friends, they reassured me that boys often developed slower than girls, and I shouldn't compare. I made a note to check with his doctor at Caleb's upcoming immunization visit. On examination day, the pediatrician took a double take at the scans and exclaimed, "I cannot believe these scans go with this kid!" He told me he saw nothing wrong with him and that in every way he seemed perfectly normal. I shrugged off my concerns.

By seven months, Anna Catherine's records showed her standing against things and "cruising." At seven months, Caleb could only lie there when placed on his stomach. During the middle of his 8th month, he started creeping in an army style movement. He would use his left side to propel his body forward and literally drag his right side on his stomach. At least he was moving, but it was obvious there was a major problem with the right side.

When he was 11 months old, I wrote a prayer letter to my team. I listed the things he could do and then I told of the things he couldn't do and how that made me feel. Below is the letter.

*** HE CAN NOT***

*** He can't crawl on all fours*
*** He can't wave or say bye bye*
*** He can't clap his hands together*
*** He can't get to sitting position from the floor*
*** He can't bang objects with his right hand (like he will take a spoon and bang a pot with his left but even if we physically hold his right hand and force it to hit, he fights it.*
*** He doesn't seem to get "no". By this age, a.c. would look at you with this sly little look before she did something she knew she shouldn't. Caleb has never done that although there are PLENTY of things we say NO to. (This is a concern since his right frontal lobe is gone, which has the ability to discern right from wrong)*

It is very obvious that his left side is BY FAR dominant. They told us that due to the extensive brain damage on his left side, his right side may not have any purposeful movements. He definitely can use it purposefully but not naturally (meaning normally he just clinches that fist unless we do something to force him to use it).

These are the facts. Now, let me try and share with you my thoughts, prayer request, etc.

76

First of all, let me reiterate that Percy and I both feel strongly that God told us he would heal Caleb. I still feel that deep in my soul... that he is healed... that he will live a normal life.

BUT... there are days like last night when I just start crying. Last night, I was adding some videos to my computer and accidentally hit on a video of Anna Catherine when she was 9 months old (2 mo. younger than Caleb right now). She was walking, dancing, babbling, laughing and saying bye bye with a wave of her hand.

Most days I force myself not to compare the two because I know Anna Catherine was advanced. But last night I just suddenly started crying and thought "what if I am just in denial?" How long can I play the "well, I can't compare because all kids are different" game? At some point, I may just have to say Caleb is not normal. Or maybe I am leaning too much on the supernatural and not doing enough on my own. Yes, God says He heals but that doesn't mean medicine and therapy don't have a place in that.

I vacillate back and forth saying "Ashley, you are exaggerating the problem. So he can't wave bye. I am sure other normal kids don't do that at ten months. So, he isn't crawling. I am sure other kids that are normal don't do that"...etc., to the point that I treat Caleb totally normal and do nothing about any potential disabilities, telling myself they are so small it is probably my imagination.

OR, I feel like I am feeling today. I feel a great pressure to find exercises I can do with him. I wish I could get him examined by a neuro-psychologist who could really see if there are some warning signs and if there are things I can do now with his young impressionable mind to fix things.

I met a lady who has a daughter with brain damage here in my neighborhood. She goes every six months to Philadelphia to this place called "The Institutes". Her daughter was supposed to be a vegetable and now at five years is crawling and starting to talk. She is so amazed at the things they know how to do now to treat brain injuries. She gave me a book by the founder, Glenn Doman, called "What to do about your brain injured Child". I am also fascinated with all the treatments one can do.

Again I waver... am I being a bad parent for not seeking these things out? Should we go to the states for an evaluation at this place? Should we be traveling 5-6 hours down to South Africa every month to meet with specialist doctors than aren't available here in Botswana? This lady has employed two ladies to help with doing different exercises and therapies all day with her child. Should I do that? Am I being *cheap for saying that all this costs ALOT of money and we just can't afford that? Or is this the kind of thing that involves your child and you will eat beans and rice to make sure your child gets the best treatment?*

OR, is this the kind of thing I need to spend more time in prayer claiming his healing. Should my belief in Caleb's healing lead me to do therapies with Caleb but not to spend our savings or rearrange our entire lives to try and treat something which may not be a big deal anyway?

I constantly wonder what the line is between walking in faith and being a responsible parent.

I wrote that email on Thursday, July 29. Later that day, a lady from Johannesburg wrote and encouraged me to visit an occupational therapist there. I laughed thinking how easy she made it sound to just jump in a car and go to South Africa. It was around a 5 hour drive, not counting the time spent at the border, which was totally unpredictable depending on the day. Percy would have to take off at least two work days, and his leave days were valuable and few. Fuel was expensive; hotel costs were through the roof in the big metropolitan city and food costs were high. Then, there was just the pure headache of travelling long distances with two small children in the car and sleeping together in one hotel room. The more I thought about it, the more convinced I became that a trip to Johannesburg was out of the question.

Friday, July 30th, Percy came home and told me he had bad news. He had just found out he had to go to Johannesburg the next week. He began to apologize, knowing I always hated to be left alone with the kids for long periods of time. Mid sentence he stopped as he saw my face light up. I never got excited when he told me he had business trips! What was wrong with me he wanted to know? My head was spinning. Wheels were churning! Could this be an opportunity to accompany Percy and take Caleb for a complete assessment with an experienced child therapist?

It was a long shot with lots of hurdles to leap over. I mentally ran through the hurdle list. Percy's boss would have to approve Caleb and me accompanying Percy in the car as well as the hotel room. Today was Friday. Percy left on Monday; how was I going to find a therapist with an open slot on such short notice? Percy would be at meetings all day, unavailable to help with transport. In addition, it would really be better to not go with two kids. Who could keep Anna Catherine at a moment's notice?

We started with his boss. Percy asked if we could accompany him in the car and in the hotel if we were willing to pay the difference of the double occupancy. His boss said no need to pay the extra money and didn't mind at all if we went! One hurdle down... lots more to go! Finding Anna Catherine a babysitter went smoothly also. Dana's family, the one who had previously kept her, said it would be their pleasure to have her again. Next, I began calling different therapists. One was booked; another one could see me but needed a follow up appointment to discuss her advice.

Finding an O.T. looked like the snag until one lady suggested a friend of hers who was on maternity leave. It was a lot to expect a new mother to come in to the office and do a favor for a complete stranger. I explained our situation, our limited time in Johannesburg, and told her Caleb's history. To my surprise, she said she would be glad to see us. Her only condition was that she couldn't make a specific appointment time until that day because she would need to schedule around her baby's feeding times. No problem, I had nothing else on my agenda but to see her.

There was one more hurdle to go – transportation. I had to find a ride to get to her. I called a few people but they all voiced their apologies for one reason or another. I had held off calling the Randolph's, the couple who had waited for us on the day we got the first brain scans. They had been so helpful during our lengthy hospital stay. They had bought extra change of clothes, a computer, picked up my parents from the airport, and even visited regularly. When we went to Pretoria, we had not known their names. By the time we left, we felt forever indebted to them for their kindness and hated asking them for another favor. But, my options had run out; they were my last hope. To my relief, they were delighted to assist once again and so was I! What a blessing friends from the Lord were!

Within a couple of hours, I had a whole trip to South Africa planned and it looked like our only expense was going to be my food and the O.T. appointment! I couldn't stop smiling at God's goodness to us!

When I made the appointment with the O.T., I explained Caleb's history and brain damage. I walked in straddling Caleb on my hip; she looked behind me as if expecting someone else. I turned as well but saw no one. I asked if we should wait for someone else. She looked at me inquisitively, cocked her head, and asked with a puzzled look on her face, "Is that Caleb?" I nodded yes and we followed her into a room.

The first thing she did was start packing toys and tests. She exclaimed, "Well, I guess we won't need any of these! When you said brain damaged, I was picturing a very different scenario!" She reached for my scans as if needing proof of my credibility. After studying them carefully, we added one more member to the "Astonished Physician's Club"!

Caleb was all giggles and smiles throughout the one hour and forty five minute session. She kept commenting on his happy, responsive disposition. "A rarity," she insisted, obviously very impressed, "in my sessions, babies are not usually this cheerful and cooperative!" On a further note, due to his right frontal lobe damage, she expected to see a volatile and irritable baby. She was truly amazed.

After a series of tests, she concluded that her main area of concern was Caleb's right side. She also noted that he lacked initiative to use it purposefully. However, in all honesty, she'd treated kids who had nothing wrong with their brains who were worse than Caleb. She also reminded me his left side was totally on par for his age. She gave me some ideas for exercises to strengthen his right side but admitted that even without therapy, he was probably going to turn out just fine!

Finally, she joined the other doctors in warning me that due to his frontal lobe damage we needed be watchful for an inability to concentrate, memory loss, and discernment of right from wrong. Like the neurologist, she agreed we wouldn't know the extent of that damage until much later. The occupation therapist did, however, positively observe that he sustained her eye contact, indicating prolonged concentration. Also, in some of her test, she'd do an action, such as banging two blocks together. Aferwards, he was asked to repeat. His ability to imitate her actions showed memory and concentration. He was right on track. Overall, she was beyond impressed and thanked me for the opportunity to work with such a good patient. His smiles had made her day!

She promised to research some good exercises to recommend for Caleb and email them to me. Goodbyes and thanks were exchanged and we were on our way. On the way home, Percy and I analyzed whether the trip was a good decision. Mark 9:24 tells the story of a man who asked Jesus if he could heal his son. The man immediately exclaimed, "I do believe; help me overcome my unbelief!" I definitely could relate to the story. The trip was a merciful gift from

God to help me overcome my unbelief. Sadly, I related too much with doubting Thomas. I needed to see the proof. I needed more than God's word at that time. I needed an unbiased professional to get that shocked look on their face and say "WOW" to spur me along in my journey of faith.

Percy dug deeper and asked about another one of my struggles. He wanted us to tackle the question of the line between totally trusting God (doing nothing to help Caleb medically) to totally revolving our lives around helping him. Sometimes I felt guilty for wanting to do exercises with Caleb all day, to get him to the best doctors, and to read the latest books on brain damage. Why, after all, did I need to do all of that if God had truly healed him? Did it show a lack of faith?

As the discussion evolved, something hit me. When we did some of the advised exercises, we could see relatively instant results. Those were just exercises that I, a mere human, could do. Caleb literally lacked the brain to communicate with his body parts in order to do these activities. God's part was making those therapies I did with Caleb achieve their desired result. The bottom line was I had to trust God for the supernatural healing.

I also started thinking about how I asked God for good health, but I still demonstrated good stewardship by eating right and exercising. So why should I feel it was a lack of faith on my part to help Caleb exercise weak parts of his body?

Finally, I understood my course of action. I was free to do the suggested exercises with Caleb, but God's healing wasn't conditional on anything I could or would do. It wasn't by works but by the Spirit of God! God had given me the calling to be Caleb's mom. With that came some added responsibilities, but I was still Anna Catherine's mom. I was still Percy's wife. I was still called to be a witness and light in my neighborhood. And, I was still called to be a missionary in our church and home. In believing God's healing promises, I had freedom to not feel guilty if my life didn't revolve around treating Caleb.

The day we got back to Botswana, Caleb started pulling up to a standing position on his own. By the next week, he was crawling on all fours like any normal baby. I hadn't even gotten the email with the occupational therapist's suggestions for exercises. I felt like God was smiling down at me and reminding me that He was healing Caleb, but in His time. I smiled back and said thanks!

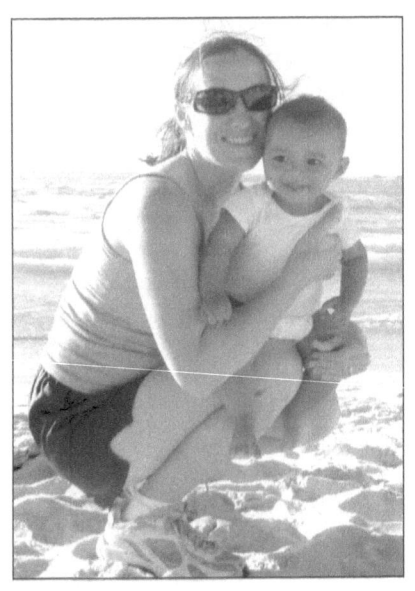
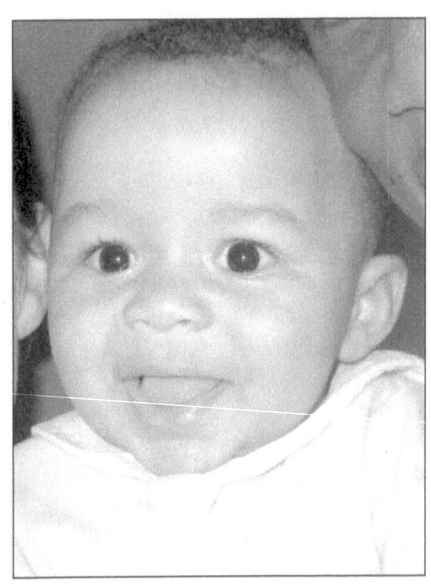

Caleb in Cape Town

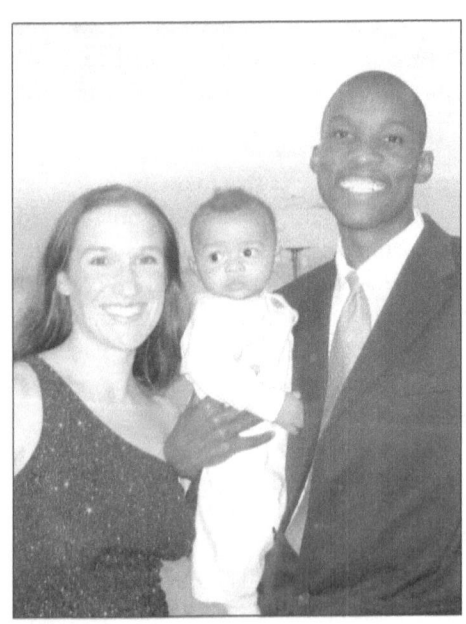
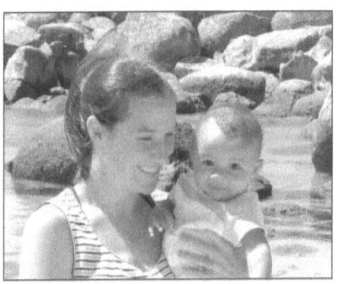
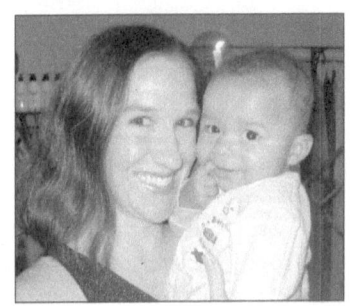

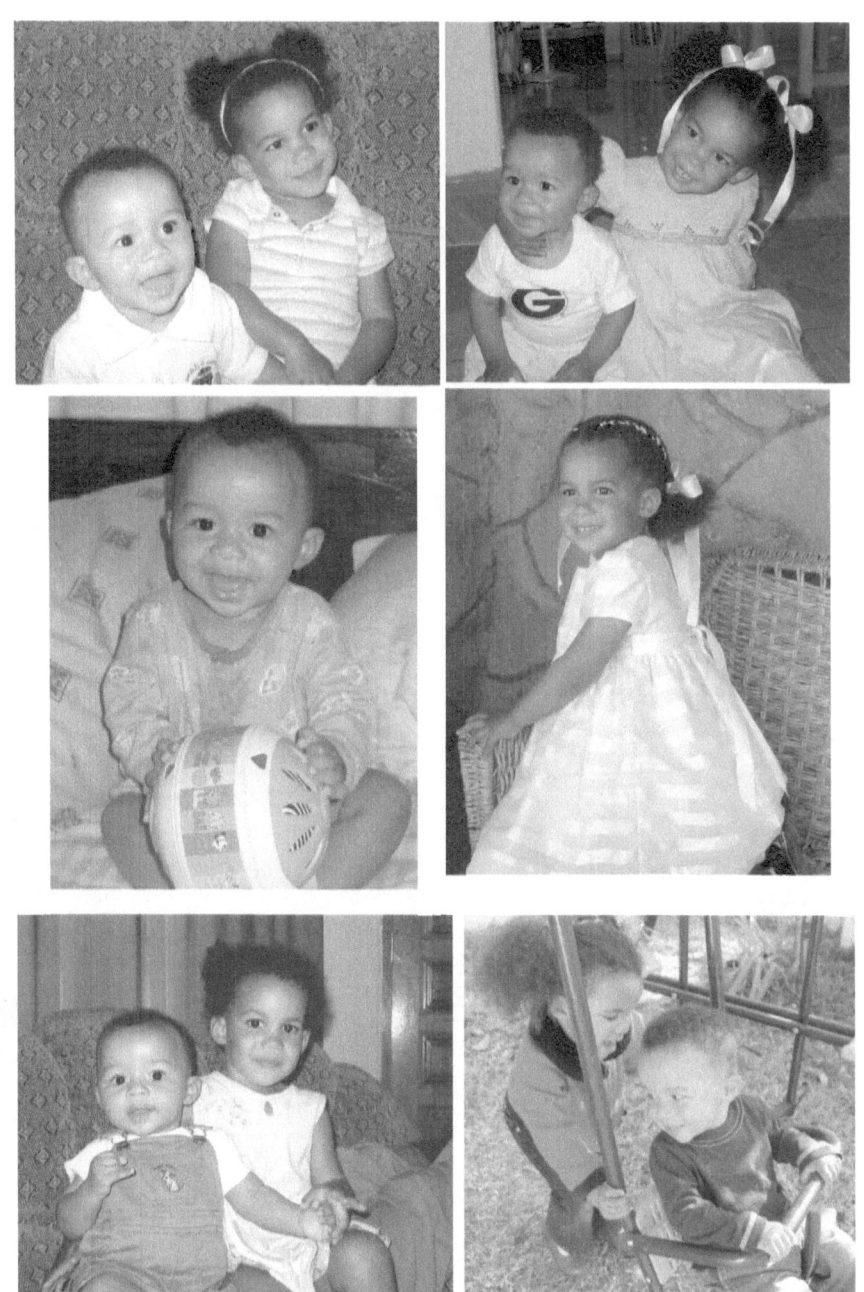

Chapter Fifteen

The not so glamorous mission field

Although my journey with Caleb brought me many smiles and taught me countless lessons, it wasn't all roses. My life was forced to revolve around my kids, and I felt trapped sometimes. This wasn't how I envisioned my life when I was growing up and dreamed of the missionary life in Africa.

I thought back to how I felt when Percy and I had moved back to Botswana with Anna Catherine. We had boarded the plane, with fresh memories of my dad's tears at the airport bidding his only granddaughter goodbye. Although I was sad to say goodbye to my parents, I could barely contain my excitement! Visions of Percy and me, as a team, leading Batswana to walk in obedience with our wonderful Lord filled my mind. We couldn't wait to tell them of the magnificent plan God had for their lives if they would turn to Him and trust His path. Oh, how we desired Batswana to know their Creator cared for them. Even if they had never experienced the love of an earthly father, they had a heavenly Father who knew them by name and was willing to die for them he loved them so much. We were excited to tell those we met that Jesus had power over fear and came to set them free from any fears they might have: fears of getting poor grades, fears of losing their job or not being successful, and fears of getting sick. He was the true Protector. No one needed to sacrifice a month's wages to a traditional doctor for immunity from harm's way. I wanted to explain that though it may make logical sense to follow their own desires that choosing to follow God's word would always lead them to an abundant life with no regrets.

Botswana has one of the highest rates of HIV positive people in the world. Some statistics put the rate as high as one in three people being HIV positive. I didn't know the exact numbers, but I knew for sure it was a major problem. Sadly, story after story seemed to convey that the main cause of this rapidly spreading pandemic was sex before marriage with multiple partners or affairs within marriage. We wanted to share how God's word and His Spirit within us continually gave us the strength to remain faithful to each other. We wanted to share with young couples practical tips on how their marriages could bring them happiness and fulfillment and last a lifetime. We wanted to testify to the joy we had knowing that we had saved ourselves sexually until marriage. We wanted them to know that purity was possible and bear witness that faithfulness brought trust and love into relationships. OH! Percy and I were so excited! We couldn't wait to start our ministry. Surely God had great plans in store to give us such an assurance that this move was His will.

Two months after our arrival in Botswana, we were still jobless and moving from house to house as different people asked us to housesit or visit. But our prayers didn't change. We were so sure of God's call that we were able to THANK Him for His goodness in His provisions within our lives. However, there was one thing I was starting to get discouraged about. I was basically just sitting at home. Sure, I was trying to hit the streets and reach the nations with the good news about Jesus! But with Anna Catherine's nap times, it was difficult to even get out. When I did, my little girl ended up demanding most of my attention so life changing conversations were hard to come by!

Life settled in place, Percy was swamped working nearly 60-70 hours a week and I became a stay at home mom. Where was the glamorous mission field I had once known? In its place were dirty diapers, a little girl that needed constant entertainment, and a very tired, bored mom.

Weeks turned into months. Months turned into years. I started some home Bible studies, did some neighborhood evangelism, and together, we worked with a couple of local church ministries. Activity was slim, but God was working and even blessed me with the opportunity to see a few people decide to follow Him for eternity. It just didn't seem enough! I wanted that sense of fulfillment from spending my days reaching out to the masses! I felt like a prisoner in my own home. When I complained to Percy, he asked if I should try and get a job and hire a nanny. No, I knew that at this point in my life I was called to be home with my little girl.

"Then," he asked, "Why are you complaining if you know that this is what you are supposed to be doing?"

"Yes, this may be what God has planned for me, but it doesn't mean I like it," I whined! For the first time in my life, the job I knew God was calling me to do didn't bring that inner sense of satisfaction and constant joy! As a full time missionary, I got excited listening to people's testimonies and seeing lives changed for the better. As a mother, I got excited that I had managed to cook dinner with Anna Catherine hanging on my leg! I could be doing the housewife thing at home in the comforts of America! I could be doing the mom job with my parents just down the street to share in the joy of my beautiful daughter.

I still was confident God had called me back to Africa, but why?

I didn't have the answer, just more questions. If I thought I was a "prisoner" as a mother of one, it certainly didn't get better when Caleb entered the picture. Any mom who has multiple small children knows that just a trip to the grocery store becomes an all day affair! It is even harder with some of the challenges I encounter living in Botswana: having to go to three stores to find just half of the ordinary items on my grocery list, poor customer service, swipe machines not working and having to run to the ATM holding two kids, etc. Countless times I pondered, isn't there more to God's plan for my life than this?

In the meantime, with as much passion and excellence I could muster, I tried to fulfill God's calling. Anna Catherine learned to pray, and we began to pray for people by name on our street. The children and I read Bible Stories while I taught Anna Catherine her alphabet letters. Anna Catherine and I had many "training" sessions on love and sharing, while she struggled to share my attention with Caleb. She could pitch quite the fit because she had become used to having all my time.

I tried to take my negative thoughts captive and make them obedient to Christ. I sought to dwell on things that were lovely and true so that I could be a happier wife for Percy to come home to and a more positive follower of Christ in general.

Below is a prayer letter I wrote expressing some of my motherly woes:

On a personal note, I would like to share with you what has been consuming much of my prayer life now.

Entering into the New Year, very aware of the absence of a Christmas holiday with my family (in the States), I am reminded again that I live in a foreign land. Every time Caleb giggles, rolls over, tries to sit up, etc. I can only write about that to my parents. Each time Anna Catherine does something to make us smile, I come face to face with the reality that my parents will never really get to experience my wonderful children growing up, I am reminded that I am a missionary in a foreign land. I say all this to say that I am

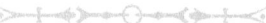

daily reminded of what I am missing out on raising my children in a distant land; BUT I KNOW that God called me here and even through the sadness this reality brings, there is a peace that I know I am where God wants me to be. He called me to Botswana.

NOW, the prayer request... So, what does that mean to be the "mom and wife" and "the missionary?" I could have easily just been a stay at home mom and raised my kids in the States so I don't want to just get comfortable being a "stay at home mom" here in Botswana and not get out in the "fields." Yet I struggle some days to muster the energy to plan ministry events and reach out to others. I am lucky now because most afternoons, there is a time of about an hour where their nap times overlap and I get some peace and quiet. It is during this time that I can host bible studies, do my quiet time to prepare for bible studies, prepare food for others, etc. Some days, my Spirit is soo willing to just take that time and read my Bible and pray for the people God has laid in my path, or invite someone over during that time with the purpose of reaching out to them, etc., but my flesh says "take a nap!" "just chill and read a book".. and it is so easy to fall into a complacent role of just staying at home all day... raising the kids and relaxing when they sleep. BUT, I want my life to count!!! I don't want to say I left my family just to chill here in my house in Africa! Soooo.... pray for me that I would have the energy to be intentional about living each day to the fullest!!! :)

Now, with that said, the opposite also happens. I have seen there have been times here when I volunteer to do so much that the kids' nap times suffer, they get ignored, they end up eating cookies and junk for meals because I didn't have time to cook, etc. as I serve others. Having been in full time ministry for so long, it is hard to not use "full time" as the standard to what I feel like I need to be doing. I have to realize that I am not full time right now... my husband works all day and that leaves me in charge of raising our children. I have to realize that in and of itself is a ministry not to be shrugged off. But, sometimes that job feels not as glamorous as being out there reaching the masses for Jesus, but I wanted to share with you a wakeup call I had this morning that brought me to tears remembering again the great role of a parent.

I was told this morning at church of a boy who wanted an expensive cell phone. He wanted to fit in with his friends so badly. His father refused. He took a belt and hung himself. He was dead by the next day. They buried him this morning before church. In his 14-year-old mind, if he couldn't have what all his other friends had, life wasn't worth living!

I have a great responsibility to truly teach my children that their worth is in Christ not in the approval of others, the material things of this world, or even in the good and bad things life throws at us. Suicide in teenagers here is unbelievably high.

Usually it is related to bad grades, a romantic relationship gone sour, or AIDS... but the point is ending one's life is a very popular answer to dealing with problems over here. My children will need to know that is not an option. We serve a God who will walk with us through any valley and is our present help in any circumstance.

Please pray for me. I want so badly to be a light outside of my home and I feel God called me here to Botswana to be just that. However, pray for me as I am equally called to be a light INSIDE my home. I want a balance that gives me peace and purpose.

Thank you as always for walking with us and praying for us!! Thankful also that in Christ we are pressed but not crushed, persecuted but not abandoned, struck down but never destroyed!!!! Though our sorrows may last for a night, in Christ, JOY comes in the morning!

Ashley :)

Don't get me wrong, I truly loved my kids and knew that I was blessed to be able to stay at home with them all day. Nevertheless, I constantly wondered why my African ministry seemed to be only affecting a handful of people when I truly thought God had a plan to use me to be a blessing to many.

September 5, 2010 rolled around and I realized it was only two days before my baby boy turned one! So many people had been faithful to pray for Caleb without the chance of ever meeting him. The idea of a video popped into my heard as the perfect praise report. I spent almost a whole day filing through a year's worth of video footage of Caleb. Eventually, I trimmed it to a 5 minute YouTube clip, capturing his major milestones throughout his first year. (The video link is: **http://www.youtube.com/watch?v=T4kmQXuaonE&feature=mfu_in_ order&list=UL**) It took 26.5 hours to upload with our tortoise speed internet. Finally finished, my prayer team and a few of their connections could view Caleb's story.

To my shock, within one week over 1400 people had watched it. Emails streamed in by the hundreds. People from all walks of life shared how Caleb's story had strengthened their faith. A doctor verified that it was the most authentic miracle he had experienced in over 47 years of medical practice. A nurse humbly admitted to struggling as she had followed our story, wondering why God would allow such an awful thing to happen to an innocent baby. Seeing this video convinced her that God had a plan all along. A friend had renewed her desire to pray, and was amazed that God actually answered her prayers. Countless mothers wrote, saying that watching and listening to Caleb's story had made them count their blessings for their healthy kids. Pastors asked permission to show the video in their Sunday morning "testimony slot". Surprisingly, one lady even wrote, "You are the talk and rejoicing of this town, at Bible study, water aerobics, around town, if someone didn't get the video, they want it. God is sooooo good!"

As the emails and facebook comments kept trickling into my inbox, I sat in awe. I had questioned God. I had thought he wanted to use me to be a blessing to others. In my limited mind, that meant physically going out and sharing His magnificent plan with people explaining how they could repent of their sins and choose to follow the One who knew every thought in their minds and hair on their heads and had a wonderful plan for their lives. If I had done things my way, maybe 50-100 people would have been reached …maybe! I am amazed to say that I honestly have no idea how many lives have been touched and encouraged through Caleb's story! And that has nothing to do with me! I have simply shared my observations in watching God work in Caleb's life from my front-row seat as his mother!

I was humbled as I felt like God looked down at me and said, "oh, ye of little faith. I told you I had a plan! All those hours you sat loving, praying for, and nurturing your son in the privacy of your home when no one but me watched, I was using you. You had your boxed-in plans, but what I had in mind was far greater than you could have ever imagined. "Mark 9:36-38 says, *"36He took a little child and had him stand among them. Taking him in his arms, He said to them, 37"Whoever welcomes one of these little children in my name welcomes me; and whoever welcomes me does not welcome me but the one who sent me."*

I had been looking all over to see where God was working, overlooking the obvious… in the very ministry that came so naturally –the role of a mother. I was filled with a renewed desire to welcome HIS plan (in whatever shape or form that may come) and depend on Him to fill in the pages of my life story. Truly, as the old song says, there was no other way to be happy in Jesus, but to trust and obey!

The video link is:

http://www.youtube.com/watch?v=T4kmQXuaonE&feature=mfu_
in_order&list=UL

The kids that keep me so busy

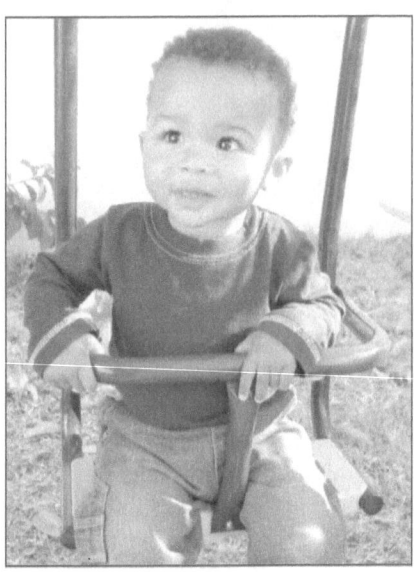

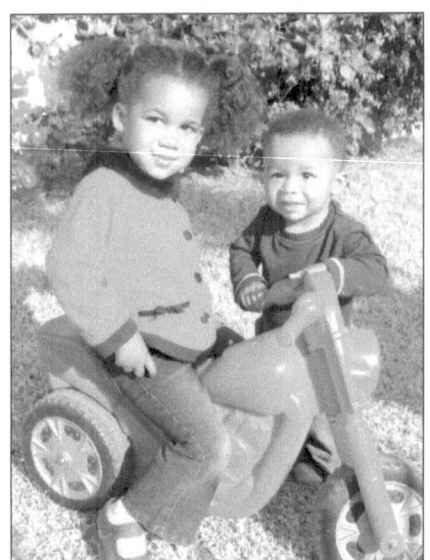

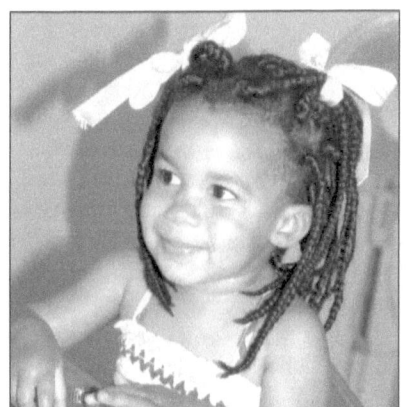

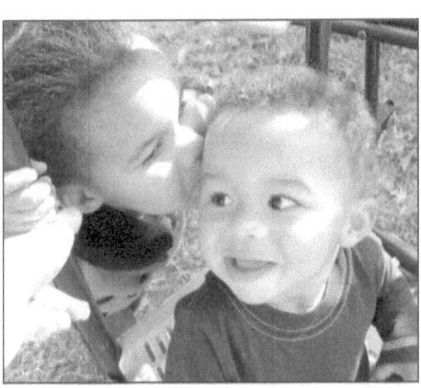

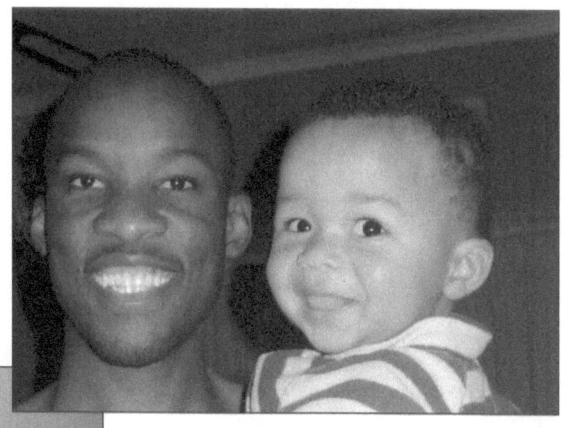

Daddy's little boy

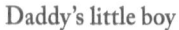

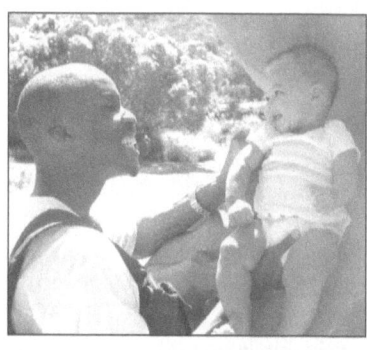

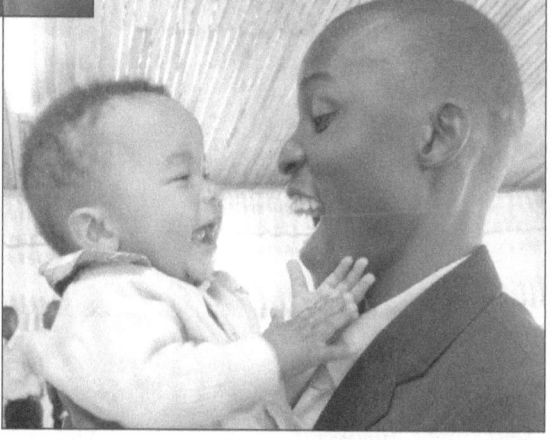

Chapter Sixteen

He who began a good work will complete it

Over the past year, well-meaning friends, in love, have said things like the following: "Oh, if you had just gone to South Africa in the beginning, none of this would have happened."

"This probably wouldn't have happened in America; it is really too bad that you chose to deliver in Botswana".

"I am so sorry that this had to happen to you."

As I close this book, I reflect on these statements. In all honesty, healthy deliveries occur every day in Botswana; medical tragedies happen in every country of the world. This could have happened anywhere. It is true, however, that if Caleb had been born with no complications, it would have saved us A LOT of tears and grief! YET, it would have kept us from knowing so many valuable lessons that could never have been learned sitting in a church or a morning quiet time in the coziness of our home.

We learned that there is NOTHING we can't get through when God gives us strength. We learned that His power IS greater in our weakness! ALL things DO work together for the good of those who love the Lord. He is faithful to take care of ALL of our needs when we seek Him first! We discovered first hand that He will walk with us through the valley of the shadow of death! We learned the power of prayer, the POWER OF GOD!

We had never felt such love, such support, and such a tangible feeling of being lifted up to the throne of God by saints praying for us around the world! We were stunned at how many friends we had!

Would I have done things differently if I had known how badly things would go in Botswana? Probably. I can't imagine choosing that kind of trauma for a helpless infant. But, do I have any regrets? NO! I am so thankful that I gave God my life and chose to trust Him, in His sovereignty, to guide me to an abundant life. This was not the path I would have chosen for myself. Yet, God, in His infinite wisdom, knew this circumstance was just what I needed to draw me close to Him and to bring glory to His name worldwide!

As I write this, Caleb is still young. Medically, we are not out of the "woods" yet. They predict due to his right frontal lobe basically being destroyed that he will have many social problems as he matures. However, we are confident in this. He who began a good work in our son will carry it to completion! We choose to believe, and we choose to praise God in faith for we KNOW He is a GOOD GOD and our loving Father!!

I don't know what you are going through in your life right now. Maybe you are walking down a path that you would have never chosen for yourself. Let me encourage you to stop and seek God. Find a quiet place and pull out your Bible and let His words become a balm to your aching soul. Meditate on His promises until you actually believe they are true! Choose to praise God and thank Him for that which is good in your life. Don't allow yourself to be consumed with the negative things surrounding you.

He came to give us an abundant life! Seek Him first, and I can personally attest that He will take care of your needs. He has plans to prosper you and not to harm you! He says trust in Him and lean not on your own understanding; in all your ways, acknowledge Him and He will direct your path!

We serve a mighty God, a loving God who is close to us when we are in trouble. We serve a God whose hand is not too short to save. NOTHING is too hard for the God we serve!

All that is praiseworthy will be found as we daily choose to rest in Him! Apart from Him we can do nothing, nor will we ever find the joy, peace, and love we were created to experience! Apart from Him, we will miss out living an amazing adventure story that even the best author could ever write!

Our Creator calls. He lovingly beckons us. Our Friend and Father tells us the great and unsearchable things we want to know. Our healer feels our pain. Our redeemer wants to make something out of our life that will last for eternity. Our adoring Savior wants to save each of us, his carefully planned creations, even today.

Will you trust Him and join me in praising God? Maybe your life experiences will be the next glorious story I read!

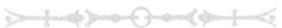

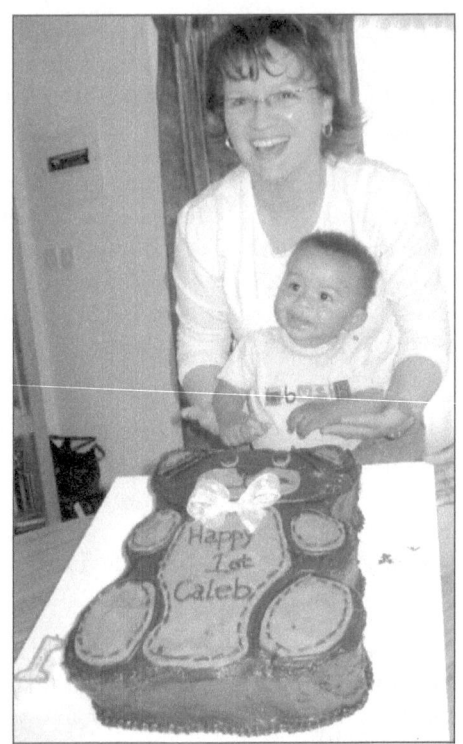

Dana, the lady who kept A.C. while we were in the hospital, made Caleb a cake for his first birthday.

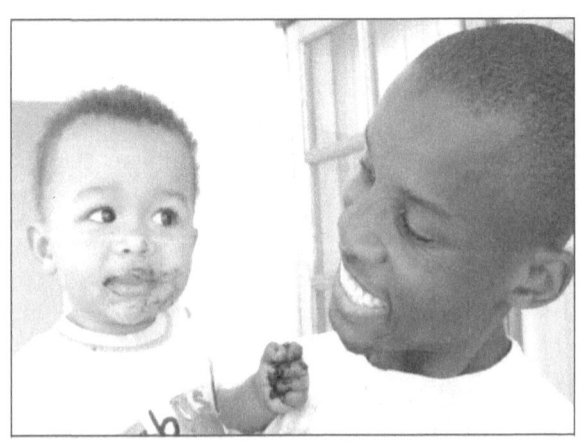

Caleb's face and hands after eating the cake

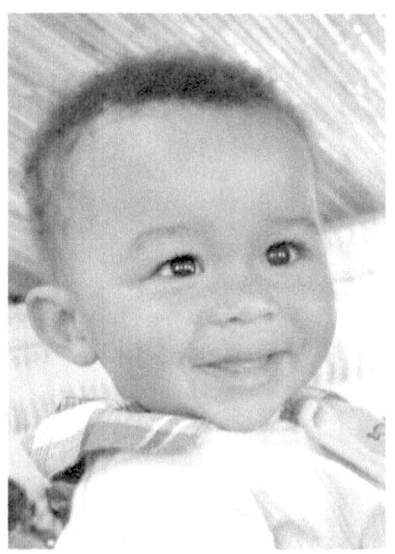
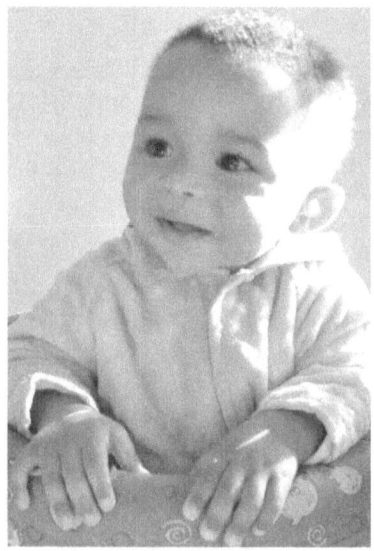

Author's note

I wrote this book in hopes that you would be able to relate with a piece of my story and be encouraged in your walk with God. Perhaps you have been wronged by someone. Whether it was their desire to hurt you or an accident, it doesn't matter to you; their actions are causing you to harbor bitterness within your heart which is preventing you from living in peace. I pray that Caleb's story will challenge you to forgive those who have wronged you and free you of the heavy load you carry. Perhaps someone you love has been given a grim medical prognosis and you are asking where God is in your pain. I pray that Caleb's story will give you hope. Perhaps you also have felt God promising healing but have yet to see the physical manifestations and are losing faith. Again, I empathize with you and say, let's walk in faith and not by sight and claim God's promises are yes and amen in Christ!

Perhaps you are the Christian housewife that wonders what her purpose is and feels bored and lonely. Let's know that God sees us and has a plan for us and work as if working for the Lord, with cheerfulness, knowing all things work together for the good for those who love the Lord.

Perhaps you don't believe that God truly loves you and cares about you personally. Perhaps you think that God is too busy to be concerned with your problems since He has the whole world to run. I hope my testimony will bear witness that God desires to be intimately involved with every detail of our lives if we will invite Him in.

I promise you that choosing a relationship with God is the most awesome decision you will ever make. The Bible says in Jeremiah 29:11-13 that God has plans to prosper you and not to harm you IF you seek God first. The Bible tells you that you don't have to worry about tomorrow IF you seek God first. If you decide to let God be the master of your life and hand over control to Him, He will lead you to an abundant life. After all, He did create life; it would make sense that He would know the best way to live it!

If you would like to have a relationship with God and have questions, I encourage you to find a Bible believing church. If you don't know how to find one or maybe you are shy to ask your questions to strangers, feel free to email me and I will see if I can help. My email is *ashleythaba@gmail.com*

Also, *if you would like to know how to get more copies of the book*, please email me as well and I can arrange to get you more books.

Thank you for reading Caleb's story.

I hope you were blessed! ☺

www.ingramcontent.com/pod-product-compliance
Lightning Source LLC
Chambersburg PA
CBHW020927180526
45163CB00007B/2912